Pain and its Relief in Childbirth

The Results of a National Survey conducted by the National Birthday Trust

For Churchill Livingstone:

Publisher: Peter Richardson
Project Editor: Lucy Gardner
Copy Editor: Neil Pakenham-Walsh
Production Controller: Neil Dickson

Pain and its Relief in Childbirth
The Results of a National Survey Conducted by the National Birthday Trust

Edited by

Geoffrey Chamberlain MD FRCS FRCOG FACOG (Hon)
Professor of Obstetrics and Gynaecology,
St George's Hospital Medical School, London, UK

Ann Wraight RGN RM MTD
Research Midwife, National Birthday Trust;
Midwife, St George's Hospital Medical School, London, UK

Philip Steer BSc MD FRCOG
Professor and Head of Department,
Academic Department of Obstetrics and Gynaecology,
Charing Cross and Westminster Medical School, London, UK

Foreword by
Margaret Brain OBE RGN RM MTD FRCOG
President of the Royal College of Midwives, London, UK

CHURCHILL LIVINGSTONE
EDINBURGH LONDON MADRID MELBOURNE NEW YORK AND TOKYO 1993

CHURCHILL LIVINGSTONE
Medical Division of Longman Group UK Limited

Distributed in the United States of America by Churchill
Livingstone Inc., 650 Avenue of the Americas, New York, N.Y.
10011, and by associated companies, branches and
representatives throughout the world.

First published 1993
  Reprinted 1994

ISBN   0-443-04658-1

British Library Cataloguing in Publication Data
A catalogue record for this book is available from
the British Library.

Library of Congress Cataloging in Publication Data
Pain and its relief in childbirth: the results of a national
  survey/conducted by the National Birthday Trust; edited by
  Geoffrey Chamberlain, Ann Wraight, Philip Steer; foreword
  by Margaret Brain.
       p.   cm.
  Includes index.
  ISBN 0-443-04658-1
  1. Anesthesia in obstetrics—England—Statistics.
2. Analgesia—England—Statistics. 3. Medical care surveys–
England—Statistics. I. Chamberlain, Geoffrey, 1930–
II. Wraight, Ann. III. Steer, Philip J. IV. National Birthday
Trust Fund (Great Britain)
     [DNLM: 1. Pain—therapy. 2. Labor. WQ 300 P144 1993]
RG732.P35   1993
617.9′682—dc
DNLM/DLC
for Library of Congress   93–20137
                                             CIP

Published by Longman Publishers Singapore Pte Ltd
Printed in Singapore

Contents

Contributors

Geoffrey Chamberlain
MD FRCS FRCOG FACOG (Hon)
Professor of Obstetrics and Gynaecology,
St George's Hospital Medical School, London,
UK

Harold Gamsu FRCP (E) FRCP DCH MB BCh
Reader in Neonatal Medicine and Consultant
Paediatrician, King's College School of Medicine
and Dentistry, London, UK

Maldwyn Morgan MB BS DA FFARCS FRCAnaesth
Reader in Anaesthetic Practice and Honorary
Consultant Anaesthetist, Royal Postgraduate
Medical School, London, UK

Ann Oakley MA PhD
Professor of Sociology and Social Policy,
University of London; Director, Social Science
Research Unit, Institute of Education, London,
UK

Philip Steer BSc MD FRCOG
Professor and Head of Department, Academic
Department of Obstetrics and Gynaecology,
Charing Cross and Westminster Medical School,
London, UK

Ann Wraight RGN RM MTD
Research Midwife, National Birthday Trust;
Midwife, St George's Hospital Medical School,
London, UK

Foreword

Audit is now becoming widespread and is even popular with midwives and doctors throughout the country. They are measuring what they do and the efficacy of their actions. They are learning from this and putting right areas they think are deficient in terms of service. Some of this is as a result of the Department of Health's efforts in promoting audit in the reformed Health Service. However one organisation has been doing such measurements of women and their birth patterns for over 50 years. The National Birthday Trust, founded between the wars, has mounted surveys on various aspects of the maternity services in order to measure what is happening in the whole country. These have usually been done on a large enough sample to give a powerful number of women and their pregnancy events. National Birthday Trust reports have been published over the years and taught professionals, managers and the public much about current trends.

The latest of these surveys is reported in this volume. A study was done by the National Birthday Trust to examine carefully the use of pain relief in childbirth. A senior midwife and two professors of obstetrics ran the national survey in 1990 which examined in detail the method of pain relief being planned and used as well as the results. This survey was unique in that it assessed the effect of the woman's pain relief from three points of view obtaining answers from the mother herself, her partner (if he was present) and the midwife. Since virtually everybody in this country is tended by a midwife and some 85% of their partners are husbands this gave a much more complete picture with three points of view of the pain relief achieved. The pattern of usage and the deficiences are shown up in this report and I recommend it as important reading for all midwives, obstetricians and anaesthetists who help women in labour. One important area is where no formal pharmacological analgaesia was offered and the woman used non-pharmacological methods of pain relief. This has been assessed carefully. Furthermore, a 6-week follow up of reactions to pain at a later stage makes this an important study.

The National Birthday Trust is soon to combine with the charity Birthright. We, as midwives, hope that it will continue its work performing socio-epidemiological measures to keep us informed of what we are doing and thus help us all improve our practice.

1993   Margaret Brain

Preface

The National Birthday Trust is a charity concerned with the care of women and their babies around the time of childbirth. In 1990, a survey assessed pain in labour and the techniques of analgesia throughout the United Kingdom. The Trust now publishes the results and some interpretations from this study, the fifth of the post-War survey analyses on maternity services.

By turning to pain relief in labour the National Birthday Trust goes back to one of its major aims at its foundation in 1928. In one week in June 1990 all deliveries in the United Kingdom were surveyed. The editors of this report have brought together the results and suggested implications from the survey data. The survey team, Ann Wraight (a midwife) and Professors Geoffrey Chamberlain and Philip Steer (obstetricians) was based at St George's Hospital and both the District Health Authority and Medical School are thanked for their generous accommodation. The Statistical Department at the School assisted with the data analysis and we are particularly grateful to Professor Martin Bland and to Dr Valerie Dickinson and Mr Richard Hulkhory from the Computer Department. The coordinators completed much of the report themselves but valuable help was given in specialist areas by members of the Birthday Trust scientific team, notably Dr Harold Gamsu (Paediatrics), Dr Maldwyn Morgan (Anaesthesia) and Professor Ann Oakley on the longer term attitudes to childbirth. The survey was funded mostly by the National Birthday Trust with a generous donation from the Department of Health to whom we are grateful. We are also appreciative of the efforts made by our publishers, Churchill Livingstone, and particularly our editor, Ms Lucy Gardner. The script was typed many times by Mrs Sarah Reed, whose patient work has led to the final results. Illustrations were produced by Duncan Larkin of the Audio-Visual Department of St George's Hospital.

This survey could not have taken place if the women and their partners had not made such a big effort to fill in the forms. The Trust is appreciative of this. Our final thanks go as always to the midwives who carried out most of the real work. The midwife in Britain is a very special person and the Trust appreciates this and is grateful to them as a body. Because of this, we have asked that the Foreword to this volume be written by the President of the Royal College of Midwives, Miss Margaret Brain.

Pain Relief in Labour Survey   Geoffrey Chamberlain
National Birthday Trust   Ann Wraight
September 1992   Philip Steer

1. The history of pain relief in labour

G. Chamberlain

Giving birth is a painful process. This applies to all social and ethnic groups and has probably been so since mankind walked upright. The stretch of the tissues at the neck of the uterus, of the vagina and of the vulva is probably the major source of pain. The contractions of the uterus going on for some hours with little relief are another source of pain, probably from tissue hypoxia. Labour pains are from deep internal organs so that as well as pain the woman has a series of intensive responses of blood pressure and breathing. Effective pain relief not only relieves the pains but also abolishes these later changes. A few women may pass through labour with little or no pain but most experience some to a moderate degree, and in some cases this is very severe.

Pain is a difficult symptom to measure; we only know about it via the signals carried through the nervous system and the woman's intellectual response to the stimulus. External measures by other observers are less sensitive for they measure the observed response of the woman to pain stimulation. Objective observations are relevant for as well as pain, many other emotions strike at the same time: anxiety, fear of the unknown and the sheer stress of the time that a labour has gone on. Each has its place in the observation of labour and in the survey described in this book we have endeavoured to look at several aspects, disentangling these complex scenes.

HISTORY OF PAIN RELIEF

Until about 150 years ago, the methods available for dealing with pain in labour were poor.

Egypt

Looking back as far as the Ebers papyrus (*c.* 1515 BC), there are descriptions of methods used to help a woman in labour but few of them could have been very effective (Bryan 1974). Some related to the distraction of the woman as when, for example, magic was used to transfer the pain: 'Say the words four times over a figurine of clay to be placed upon the forehead of the woman who is giving birth'.

Pain-relieving solutions were applied externally to the lower abdomen – incense, wine and ground-up scarab beetle, or tortoise shells. Internally, suppositories of honey, cinnamon and mint were given. Few of the extracts actually worked pharmacologically but much of the pain relief was achieved by peer support. Such evidence as we have of the management of birth in ancient history is of women in labour surrounded by many other female relatives all of whom were groaning and shrieking with the women having uterine contractions.

Greek and Roman

Pain relief continued in this same way into the Greek and Roman times, when a few more effective pharmacological agents were added such as the opiates from poppies and cannabis from hemp; their actions were known about and they were given freely to women in labour; in addition, various forms of alcohol were used. All had a depressant effect not only upon the woman but also on the fetus and must have been responsible for some babies being born who were unresponsive and did not start to breathe spontaneously. Mandragora, extracted from the mandragon root and suspended in wine, was sometimes used. This contained

1

scopolamine and caused sickness in many women as well as some degree of narcosis in the fetus and so was not very popular. It was felt by some that the woman would be made more comfortable from taking drugs which were extracted from local plants. These ranged from the possible help of 'giving the suffering mother two slices of the roots of white lily' to offering the ankle bone of a rabbit which had been killed on one of the first three Fridays of March. These analgesic attempts ranged from natural plant pharmacy to magical, but the usefulness of the latter should not be dismissed.

Dark and Middle Ages

Dating from this period are many treatises on medicine which include sections on childbirth. Women were accepted as midwives and in some cases as practitioners to look after women. Beds were reserved for childbirth in certain places, amongst the earliest of which was a refuge for the women of St Thomas, Southwark, set up by Richard (Dick) Whittington in 1423. This was the forerunner of St Thomas Hospital, now in Lambeth; it would seem that his ideas were to look after the unwed:

> The noble merchant Richard Whittington made a new Chamber with eight beds for young women who had done amiss in the hope of good amendment. He commanded that all the things that occurred in that room should be kept entirely secret under the pain of loss of livelihood. He would not shame any young woman in a way which might prove a hindrance to her marriage.
>
> (Rothon 1970)

Books of obstetrical advice were written throughout Europe going into quite considerable detail on the management of women with unusual presentations. The use of birth stools, position on the bed and even postmortem Caesarean sections were elaborated but almost nothing was said about pain relief in labour. Occasionally, for women having long labours, analgesia is mentioned but only as a part of the management of the long labour rather than dealing with the normal woman in pain, which seemed to be the expected state. There are many potions derived from herbs, trees, fruit, minerals and parts of animals; there are indeed more charms and practices of magic than drugs for pain relief in labour.

In the Trotula manuscript, written in the eleventh century and translated into English in the fifteenth century, are listed several mangements and drugs for women having uterine pain (Mason-Hohl 1940). Bleeding was considered helpful, and a plaster with hemp on the inside (vaginally) and nightshade on the outside could be applied to the abdomen. Alternatively one could wash the abdomen from the navel down to the private members with an infusion of penny royal, olivegandom, laurel leaves, calamint and mallows boiled in water and wine. After this, 'a fumigation could be made down below' of cloves, spikenard, nutmeg and galengale. The vaginal medication alternatively might be myrrh, olivanum, orgaeanum, calamint, cyprus, anise and mint. Another way of relieving pain was to apply a pot pourri in a cloth from the navel downwards; it should contain a handful each of rue, artemisia and woodworm with two ounces of camphor mashed together, powdered and boiled in wine. It was heated, wound up in a cloth and wrapped from the navel downwards. There are many other such manoeuvres recorded but the kindest seems to be 'and give her warm wine to drink in which cumin has been boiled'. The complexity of the recipes of some of these preparations reminds one of some of the Victorian antiseasickness preparations for crossing the English Channel. So tedious and detailed were these in their preparation that by the time they were perfected the boat would have arrived in France. Similarly by the time the attendants had finished making all these things to help the pain of the uterine contractions, the woman had delivered the baby.

Sir Fielding Ould (1742) recommends that:

> In a tedious labour if the spirits be much exhausted and the pains grow very short and of little or no advantage, then an opiate is of surprising service.

He equates this with the nurse introducing into the rectum her thumb to pull back the coccyx, or the index finger to give traction on the fetal jaw bone, two extremely unpleasant manoeuvres – maybe the opiates were just to cover these obstetrical first-aid endeavours.

It is interesting that the great William Smellie, probably the master of British midwifery in the early days of the eighteenth century, used to carry in his pockets spirits of hartshorn, tincture of castor and liquid laudanum in separate bottles. These compounds represented the total of his medicines in his prescribing armamentarium; probably it was the laudanum (which contains opiates) that was the most effective. John Burton of York published in 1751 a volume whose title was virtually the book's script: *Essay towards a complete new system of midwifery, theoretical and practical, together with several new improvements whereby women may be delivered in the most dangerous cases with more easy and safe position and has by any other method heretofore practised.* In it he refers to the use of opiates but, in the special case of breech labour and delivery with the aftercoming head of breech, he says:

> A proper opiate is of surprising service to the patients spirits, if in too much exhaustion the pains grow short or of little or no advantage. (Burton 1751)

All the other pharmacology relating to labour in that book is related to 'clisters' (poultices) and treatment of 'dryness of the parts'.

A popular means of distraction therapy was to make the woman move around actively; this ranged from gentle shaking to hasten the fetus, to a quite violent manhandling. Sometimes two or three large men would shake the unhappy mother-to-be backwards and forwards in her bed with great violence. In the middle ages, a ploughman was more frequently chosen for this purpose than any person for it was said 'to provide the best cure, always take the ploughman direct from the plough'. Other women were tossed in blankets or turned upside down and shaken, sometimes after being tied to a ladder. All these methods of pain relief were of little real use, although sometimes it distracted the woman so time passed and the labour proceeded.

1800 onwards

All these ideas were elaborated by the numerous midwives and accoucheurs who looked after women. Pain was considered to be an integral part of the process of childbirth. Now that we have tamed pain to some extent, people philosophise about whether labour really is painful or if the sensation of pain is only an inability to relax.

Distraction therapy by group shouting, as mentioned in early Egypt, was still quite common. Verdier quotes a French village midwife:

> In those days they used to scream, wow, did they scream. The old women used to say, 'Go on and cry so loud the whole village hears you'. (Verdier 1979)

In Victorian Britain it was generally considered to be bad form to make a fuss and it was considered important that the woman should not flinch.

Before the mid-nineteenth century there was virtually no effective and reliable pain relief. Some of the lower classes would get drunk to cope with the pain but alcohol is not a very good analgesic and indeed in some it had the effect of reducing the uterine contractions. It was not until the mid-nineteenth century that two drugs, ether and chloroform, were used for the first time in obstetrics. However, these two, joined later by nitrous oxide, were the only effective pain relief up until the mid 1940s.

ETHER AND CHLOROFORM

Ether was the first real pharmacological pain relief. In the 1840s this was known in America to be helpful for tooth extraction. Its first major use in Britain was at University College Hospital in London on 19 December 1846 for an amputation. It appeared in obstetrics only a few days later on 19 January 1847 when James Young Simpson, Professor of Midwifery at Edinburgh, used it to help a woman who needed a version extraction having been long in labour. Throughout that year Simpson continued to use ether for both normal and operative deliveries. However, the anaesthetised woman sometimes vomited and there were other risks, for example that ether would explode. In consequence, Simpson and others spent time looking for another agent; in November 1847 they tried chloroform, first on themselves; then, on 8 November, Simpson tried it to help a woman in labour. Seven days later, on 15 November, Simpson reported to the Edinburgh Medico-Chirurgical Society that chloroform was superior to ether – it was more pleasant to take, acted more rapidly, was more portable, and less inhalant was required. How many cases Simpson had collected in seven days from 8–15 November is not recorded, but it was a very sudden conversion from one inhalation anaesthetic to another.

Chloroform gave very good pain relief in labour but there was a lot of opposition from the conservatively minded. Some was from the Church where many clerics (all men) felt that women ought to have pain in childbirth:

> Chloroform is the decoy of Satan apparently offering itself to birthroom but in the end it will poison society and rob God of the deep earnest cries that arise in the time of trouble for help.

Simpson answered the arguments by contending that in Genesis 3:16 the quotation 'in sorrow shalt thou bring forth child' was actually a mistranslation of the Hebrew and that the crucial vexatious word should have been better translated as effort or stress rather than sorrow. In additon to the Church, a few medical people disagreed:

> Pain during operations is even desirable: its prevention or annihilation is for the most part hazardous to the patient. In the lying-in chamber nothing could be more true than this: pain is to the mother safety, its absence a destruction. Yet there are those bold enough to administer the vapour of ether or chloroform even at this critical junction forgetting it has been ordered that in sorrow shall she bring forth.

All Simpson's arguments were strongly reinforced when Queen Victoria used chloroform for the birth of her eighth child, Leopold, in 1853. She gave it the royal seal of approval, repeating the experience during her ninth and last delivery. The chloroform was given not by an obstetrician but by John Snow, a physician in London. He made his name separately by his epidemiological detective work when narrowing down an outbreak of typhoid to a given water pump in Soho. Being a public health physician of action, he removed the pump handle and thus effectively stopped the source of the typhoid.

The side effects of chloroform were well known. It was sometimes associated with irregular action of the heart and if much was given, there was sometimes liver damage leading to jaundice. Further, even small doses can diminish uterine contractions in both the first and second stage of labour. When it crosses the placenta to the fetus, chloroform depresses respiratory effort so that the newborn child has more difficulty starting to breathe. Despite its risks, however, chloroform was the first widely used and effective means of pain relief from the mid-nineteenth century to almost the middle of the twentieth century. Easy to administer capsules were to become available; these were slipped under a small mask and the woman could breathe chloroform to relieve herself of the worst pains of labour.

In a standard handbook of obstetric nursing by Haultain & Haig-Ferguson (1902) there is virtually nothing about pain relief in ordinary labour. Hot fomentations were applied to the perineum if labour was long. The only hint of effective analgesia is given in the following paragraph:

> Frequently the doctor gives a little chloroform at this stage. In preparation for this the nurse should see that false teeth are removed, and that the patient's head is low. A little vaseline or glycerine smeared over the nose and cheeks prevents the chloroform from blistering the skin.

All the other pages on the first and second stages relate to good nursing, but give no advice about pain relief.

'TWILIGHT SLEEP'

No real advance in analgesia in labour occurred for the rest of the nineteenth century. In the early 1900s came reports from the European continent of hypodermic analgesia given as a combination of morphine and scopolamine. The former is a powerful hypnotic and pain reliever while the latter blunts the memory; given together they induce continuous sleep and were said to be as powerful as chloroform; so their use spread rapidly. A skilled doctor had to stay in attendance so this limited their use. A small injection of each was given and as the dose of morphine began to wear off a second injection of scopolamine was given to prolong the morphine's influence. With the correct dosage, twilight sleep could last for many hours; amongst the early workers amnesia for labour was claimed in 95% of cases with brisk babies whose respiration was not depressed.

The essence of twilight sleep was individual management, with the doses of the drugs being titrated against the woman's own response. There were a few side-effects; for example, the scopolamine produced a dry mouth and women complained of thirst. Sometimes there were hallucinations but whilst the women may have needed to be reassured at the time, the delusions were not remembered. Noise and light had to be kept to a minimum, and so the woman was in a single room with darkened windows and no loud talking; indeed, the baby, once delivered, was removed from the room very swiftly for it was feared that the cries of the child might disturb the mother in her bemused state. Because of the great burden on individual doctors and midwives, various standardised protocols were attempted to make the method less labour intensive. They were never quite as good as the individual treatments. When barbiturates were invented some tried to introduce them as part of twilight sleep instead of scopolamine, but they have little analgesic effect; further, they did have a depressive effect on the baby's breathing and sometimes were associated with prolonged labour.

NITROUS OXIDE

Nitrous oxide was used widely for anaesthesia in the last century but was not used in obstetrics until the 1930s. At first it required the attendance of a special anaesthetist but equipment was devised whereby a premixed concentration of nitrous oxide and air was given. This was pioneered by Dr R J Minnitt of Liverpool who developed this equipment in 1933 aided by the National Birthday Trust (see Ch. 2). The concentrations were originally 45% nitrous oxide and 55% air; this was later altered to 50% of each. Minnitt's equipment was useful for midwives and jointly the British College of Obstetricians and Gynaecologists and the National Birthday Trust conducted a survey to assess its efficacy and use by midwives. Recommendations included an examination of the heart and lungs of the woman in late pregnancy (about 36 weeks' gestation) to assess her fitness to take this form of inhalation analgesia; such an examination was mandatory for midwife-booked deliveries for many years but has been dropped now. The nitrous oxide was self-administered by the woman through a face mask. Antenatal instruction was essential so that the woman was familiar with the techniques when she came to labour. It was important that inhalation should start as soon as a contraction was noticed; then pain relief might be expected some 20 seconds later.

The woman did not lose consciousness and many found nitrous oxide a very effective analgesic. It was slowly realised, however, that by reducing the amount of air by half, one was also reducing the amount of oxygen by the same proportion. Since air contains about 20% of oxygen, the woman using the Minnitt apparatus was only breathing about 10% of oxygen. Whilst this would not matter in a normal labour it could be important if the fetus was already compromised by a poor uteroplacental circulation. This led to the development of nitrous oxide and oxygen machines such as the Lucy Baldwin machine, named after the wife of the Prime Minister, Stanley Baldwin. Here the mixture of nitrous oxide and oxygen could be varied and preset so that a constant mixture would be used for the whole of the labour. In general, mixtures of 50% nitrous oxide and 50% oxygen were used, so overcoming the difficulty of nitrous oxide and air. These machines were very heavy and were only used in hospital units and maternity homes. They could never be carried by the midwives to the home where many deliveries were occurring in those days.

In Aberdeen, another anaesthetist, Dr Michael Tunstall, was working on the idea of premixing oxygen and nitrous oxide in liquid form under pressure. This work too was backed by the National Birthday Trust (see Ch. 2). Tunstall developed a safe mix which could be easily transported in cylinders – large ones for the hospitals and small ones for the homes. This gave the safety of a high concentration of oxygen (50%) with the efficacy of nitrous oxide. A small problem of layering of the liquids in the cylinder occurred if they were left standing for some time so a gentle rocking was required before use; at very low temperatures (below $-5°$ C) the layering was accelerated. This was extremely unlikely to happen in England and Wales but was possible in those cylinders stored outside in Scottish hospitals. Premixed nitrous oxide and oxygen (Entonox produced by British Oxygen) was first made in 1961 and is now available in all places where women have babies. It is amongst the most popular of pain relieving methods in labour and demand for it is likely to go on at least into the next century.

TRICHLORETHYLENE

Trichlorethylene (trilene) is related to chloroform; it is similiar to, and smells very like, the chemical used in dry cleaning shops. However, it is less toxic than chloroform and so efforts were made to find a way of dispensing it safely to labouring mothers. In 1943, Friedman produced a simple machine which would deliver trilene vapour at a constant concentration, enough to produce pain relief without producing unconsciousness. Until then the concentration of the active agent could be altered due to changes of temperature or the strength of a woman's respirations; the British College of Obstetricians and Gynaecologists was unhappy with its use. The National Birthday Trust persuaded the Medical Research Council and the National Physical Laboratory to examine the problem and improve the machine so that the disadvantages were overcome.

Friedman's equipment was approved using a concentration of between 0.35% and 0.5% trichlorethylene and air. The disadvantages of displacing oxygen were obviously not important at these levels but trilene did take rather longer to work compared with nitrous oxide. Inhalation would have to take place for a minute or two before pain relief was needed, compared with the seconds required for nitrous oxide. By the same token trilene was eliminated less quickly and so the analgesic effect would go on for longer. Hence a different timing pattern of administration of trilene was required compared with nitrous oxide.

Trilene was extremely useful in domiciliary deliveries because the machines were light and portable and could be carried by the midwives. However, in 1983 the then Central Midwives Board withdrew its approval for the use of trilene by midwives acting independently and now it is no longer used. It was a good analgesic to use at roughly the same level of effectiveness as nitrous oxide and oxygen.

METHOXYFLURANE AND ENFLURANE

In the last 20 years other inhalation agents have been used in an attempt to overcome the problems of slow uptake of trilene. More soluble agents such as methoxyflurane in the same concentration have the same sort of analgesic potency as trilene but there are problems with the maintenance of equipment and some fears of longer term renal damage; it is unlikely that this would occur at the concentrations and length of time methoxyflurane is used in obstetrics. Enflurane has arrived in the last decade, but has not been very popular because of the longer term drowsiness it produces.

PETHIDINE

Pethidine is the major new drug that has come into obstetrical use in the last half century; it is used under the names of Demeral or Dolantine in other parts of the world. Pethidine was developed in 1939 by the German drug industry; its rapid spread and production followed the need for self-injectable strong analgesic for front-line troops in tanks and small boats in battle. The Allies had put an effective blockade on Germany so that their supplies of opiates from the East were virtually stopped; hence pethidine developed perhaps more rapidly than it would have in peacetime. When the war finished, the British were granted the patent rights for pethidine production under the War Claims and it was released onto the British market within a year or two of the war finishing.

Pethidine was recognised as a powerful antispasmodic and analgesic. Unfortunately its first sales were not controlled and so people could buy it without prescription and started using it for recurrent spasmodic pain; one of the commonest of these is dysmenorrhoea. Sadly its addictive powers were not recognised until after this point so a population of addicts developed in the late 1940s, many of them nurses and midwives who welcomed its power but did not know of the dangers of frequent recurrent use. There is no risk of addiction if used occasionally as in the pain relief of labour. In 1949 pethidine was brought under the Dangerous Drugs Act and its use strictly regulated. It is now one of the most commonly used drugs throughout the Western world although its popularity is waning (see Ch. 6)

MORPHIA

Since early history, morphia and its associated products, morphine and heroin which were extracted from opium, were the standard pain relievers for women in labour when anything was given at all. A liquid extract was commonly given though occasionally in Europe it was prescribed as suppositories. The opiates were crudely extracted; therefore the amount of active agent in any preparation varied so that the effects were also variable. Morphia is very effective in producing pain relief but also makes the woman very drowsy; some crosses the placenta to reduce the respiratory drive of the baby.

Morphine and heroin (dihydromorphine) are still used in obstetrics particularly if a labour is expected to be long with an occipitoposterior position of the fetal head. Much of the opiate use, however, has been replaced by epidural and spinal anaesthesia, except in less well staffed or equipped units where the use of opiates still continues.

NON-PHARMACOLOGICAL METHODS

There are women who feel that they can deal with labour through natural processes, possibly by the stimulation of release of endorphins through the central nervous system. Much of this stems from Grantley Dick Read who published his philosophy in 1942 in *Revelations of child birth*. This was not his first volume, for in 1933 he had published *Natural Childbirth* but this did not receive so much publicity. Professor F J Brown of University College, London, and Joseph De Lee of Chicago took the ideas under their wings and made Dick Read acceptable to the profession. He already had many followers amongst the women having babies and so the two movements came together, the former more reluctantly than the latter, to examine the whole field of natural childbirth. In this volume we will refer to natural childbirth as non-pharmacological

pain relief. The National Childbirth Trust, a helpful organisation, have much of this in their philosophy and help women to learn about childbirth and to decide what methods of pain relief are appropriate to their individual needs.

Dick Read quotes, on the first page of his book, experiences that happened to him before the First World War. He outlines graphically how he went down Whitechapel Road on his bicycle to a confinement and how, underneath the railway arches, found a very poor home with a woman in a labour. There was, however, a quiet kindliness in the atmosphere:

> I tried to persuade my patient to let me put the mask over her face and give her some chloroform when the head appeared and the dilatation of the passages was obvious. She however, firmly but kindly refused to take this help. It was the first time in my short experience that I had ever been refused when offering chloroform... As I was about to leave some time later I asked her why it was that she would not use the mask. She shyly turned to me and said, 'It didn't hurt. It wasn't meant to, was it, doctor?'

Between this simple but honest idea ('... it wasn't meant to') and the more pragmatic approach of his professional colleagues ('Why then does it hurt?'), Dick Read ploughed a lonely furrow trying to find out why it was that some women could conduct a labour themselves without pain. His book is a discursive volume, and would occasionally tread on the feminist toes of the 1990s ('Pregnancy should be as normal for a woman as wage earning is for a man'). Basically Dick Read's hypothesis is that if women are informed and knowledgeable of what is going to happen, this will remove much of the fear and therefore pain.

Pursuit of such happiness for the mother often went in excess of what most women want in the 1990s. Dick Read considered that a Victorian family of seven to ten children would return us to the days when we would be 'swayed with a quiet and resistable goodness of true motherhood'. Again 'the man with a full quiver' and 'adequate maintenance is the peace loving worker whose presence in the community is an influence of moderation and reason'. These are the idealistic remarks of a liberal, but despite this the volume contains great sense in the helping of women towards understanding what happens in labour, both normal and abnormal. On this basis Dick Read was one of the pioneers. He was not, however, the only one; Fairburn, an early practitioner of antenatal care and the second President of the College of Obstetricians, wrote in 1924:

> Every individual patient must be treated as a problem to herself and an attempt made to quieten her fears and educate her as to what will be best for her and her child.

The idea was to help womem in labour to relax by teaching them beforehand about labour and how to cope with pain. This would remove tension; Dick Read considered that tension and fear were the factors that caused a tense cervix and therefore prolonged labour and pain. He found it resulted in giving unnecessary analgesics to half of his women. From these philosophies have developed a great number of other methods of analgesia.

Psychoprophylaxis is based upon Dick Read's ideas; it is not just a distraction technique but an educational method. Lamaze was a great exponent of full psychoprophylaxis preparation; he published in 1956 a paper showing that in two matched groups of labouring women (not randomised), the prepared group had a higher frequency of spontaneous vaginal delivery with a lower requirement for formal analgesia than did the other. The National Childbirth Trust has developed a system of relaxation and breathing exercises which depend again upon the twin pillars of education and training for labour. They were active in involving the partner in labour and it is probably due to their efforts that, by the 1990s 90% of women have a partner with them for some or all of labour. This partner is also offered education by the National Childbirth Trust as well as at other sources now. He is the greatest support for a woman for he knows her and her personality better than anybody else in the labour room.

Hypnosis has been helpful for a few women. The method goes back well into the eighteenth century but in labour it has never taken a prominent place because of the many hours of training and of the need for the trainer to be in attendance for much of labour; this is time-consuming at a time that cannot be predicted.

Acupuncture has relieved pain in many parts of the world for centuries. Its use in labour is small in

this country, but a number of women try it. The method again is time-consuming and is thought by some women to produce inconsistent results.

Transcutaneous electrical nerve stimulation (TENS) is a fairly recent addition to pain relief. It follows the publication of the gate theory of pain control by Wall in 1965 and consists of a small electrical stimulus to the skin at the site of the pain; this is usually over the lower lumbar and sacral regions. It seems to be helpful in the early stages of labour but has not been used long enough for full assessment.

Abdominal decompression was introduced by Haines from South Africa in 1959. He considered that by lifting the muscles of the anterior abdominal wall off the uterus, the organ was no longer flattened and so was allowed to orientate itself in relation to the pelvic brim; thus contractions were more effective and pain was relieved. Similarly excessive tension of the anterior abdominal wall itself would be reduced and so there would be less tension. It was popular in the 1960s but seems now to have lost its popularity for there were no cases reported in the 1990 survey.

LOCAL AND REGIONAL ANAESTHESIA

In the later days of the last century people tried applying the local anaesthetic agent cocaine to the vaginal walls to relieve pain; it did not work. An effective local anaesthetic was developed in Germany in the 1930s (nupercaine) and lignocaine followed in the 1940s. These were injected into the tissues of the lower vagina and the skin over the perineum; this technique was very effective for local pain relief but was used mostly after the event, i.e. for sewing up tears of the lower genital tract. This is now a common practice and lignocaine, a powerful local anaesthetic agent, is used prophylactically before an episiotomy or a tear (if there is warning) to numb the area. If it has not been given beforehand, it is always used after birth to give pain relief before repair takes place, and many women find relief from it.

With the wider use of operative vaginal obstetrics, regional anaesthesia was started in the early 1950s to numb the nerves as they came away from the pelvis and lower cervix, hence anaesthetic block of the pudendal nerve and the paracervical area became popular. These involved an injection, rather like the dentist uses when he gives a nerve block into the lower jaw, and usually good analgesia is produced. It depends upon the doctor localising the nerves very precisely and this was a skill acquired by many obstetricians. By the 1950s many vaginal operative deliveries were done under local pudendal or paracervical nerve blocks. Since then the other areas of regional anaesthesia (epidural and spinal blocks) have become more popular.

Regional anaesthesia usually involves the numbing of nerve roots close to the spinal canal. The most commonly used in Britain is an epidural anaesthetic, whilst in America spinal anaesthetic is widely used. The two should not be confused.

During *epidural anaesthesia* the local anaesthetic agent is introduced into the space outside the membranes that carry the spinal cord, so numbing the nerves as they flow through the epidural space and blocking sensation in the individual nerves. It can be given continuously, by leaving a fine plastic tube into the area outside the spinal cord so allowing long-term pain relief during labour.

Spinal anaesthesia on the other hand, involves an injection of local anaesthetic into the fluid that bathes the spinal cord. It is done usually as a single procedure to cover an operative delivery such as Caesarean section or forceps delivery. It cannot be used for the longer term relief of pain in labour. The first spinal anaesthetics were performed at the turn of the century and epidurals a year or two later.

At first the approach to the epidural space was via the caudal hiatus at the bottom of the sacrum. A needle was introduced behind the anus and passed up into the fatty tissue there. An injection allows local anaesthetic solution to travel up a few inches and so numbs the sacral nerves which supply the lower part of the genital tract; only a single injection was used.

Continuous epidural analgesia may have been tried in the early days of this century but it really started in 1946. Tuohy invented a malleable curved needle and Courebellio in Havana used this, passing a fine catheter into the epidural space, so that local anaesthetic could be given repeatedly or continuously. In the UK the technique was pioneered by Andrew Doughly at Kingston Hospital, Geoffrey Steele at Queen Charlotte's Hospital and Selwyn Crawford at the Birmingham Maternity Hospital. Its popularity with women has increased steadily, and despite its apparent disadvantages (see Ch. 6) it is probably the most effective form of pain relief in labour. It needs a skilled operator, i.e. a trained anaesthetist, to put it in and careful monitoring to watch for serious side-effects. Hence this powerful method is not available in hospitals with insufficient members of senior anaesthetists available. A small amount of the drug does reach the fetus but does not usually cause any serious side-effects. The extent of the chemical blockade is now much wider with the new local anaesthetic agents that have introduced.

REFERENCES

Bryan C 1974 The Papyrus Ebers.
Burton J 1751 Essay towards a complete new system of midwifery, theoretical and practical, together with several new improvements whereby women may be delivered in the most dangerous cases with more easy and safe position and has by any other method heretofore practised.
Haultain F W, Haig-Ferguson J 1902 Handbook of obstetrical nursing. Pentaned, Edinburg
Mason-Hohl E (translator) 1940 The diseases of women by Trotula. Wand Richie Press
Ould F 1742 Treatise on midwifery in three parts.
Rothon MC 1970 The medieval hospitals of England.
Verdier Y 1979 Façons de dire, façons de faire. Gallimard, Paris

FURTHER READING

Dick Read G 1942 Revelation of childbirth. William Heinemann, London
Rowland B 1981 Medieval women's guide to health. Kentucky State University Press, US
Shorter E 1984 A history of women's bodies. Penguin, London

2. Background to the survey

G. Chamberlain

The National Birthday Trust was founded after Janet Campbell had been proselytising in the Department of Health for the protection of motherhood through better antenatal and intrapartum care. In February 1928 a meeting was held in Central Hall, Westminster, where influential women spoke of the need for the care of the mother in pregnancy and labour. Lady Cynthia Colville was Lady in Waiting to the formidable Queen Mary and she read a message from Her Majesty:

> The Queen views with grave concern the continued high rate of maternal mortality. Her Majesty feels that a very real endeavour should be made to remove this reproach on our national life ... and trusts this may be achieved through the education of mothers themselves in the need for antenatal care and through a wider provision of first-rate medical and midwifery services. The Queen considers the time has come for concerted action to be taken in dealing with so pressing an evil and will await with interest the conclusions of this conference.

That year, the National Birthday Trust was founded, principally by Lady George Cholmondeley with much help from the Marchioness of Londonderry. The original aims of the Trust were:

- To make childbirth safer for mother and baby
- To promote the wider use of pain relief in labour
- To provide funds for the salaries of anaesthetists to cover maternity hospitals and for equipment for the greater improvement of pain relief.

The analgesic aspects of the Trust received a boost when Mrs Stanley Baldwin, wife of the Prime Minister, took an interest in this. At that time, while paying patients had pain relief, the vast majority of women delivering at home or in hospital were very rarely offered any help for the pain of labour.

THE NATIONAL BIRTHDAY TRUST ON PAIN RELIEF

All major aims of the National Birthday Trust have been fulfilled but the Trust had a special part to play in the development of effective analgesia in its early days in the country. It was responsible for the authorisation and distribution of capsules each containing 20 minims of chloroform. They were used by midwives and doctors for pain relief in labour, not just in the UK – the Trust sent capsules to several parts of the Empire, e.g. Kenya. Later, when chloroform was thought to have unacceptable side-effects, the Trust encouraged Dr Minnitt of Liverpool to develop nitrous oxide and air equipment which could be used by midwives. In November 1933 the Trust requested the British College of Obstetricians and Gynaecologists to investigate the use of analgesics in labour, especially their employment by midwives. At one stage over a third of such machines used in the UK had been paid for by the National Birthday Trust. Further, the Trust pioneered the much safer Lucy Baldwin nitrous oxide and oxygen machine; it was realised that, by reducing the concentration of oxygen or air to as much as half with nitrous oxide, the fetus might be at some risk of hypoxia, so gas and oxygen was used. Later, premixed oxygen and nitrous oxide cylinders (Entonox) were pioneered by Dr Michael Tunstall in Aberdeen, again with National Birthday Trust support.

When trilene came on the scene in the 1940s, it was the National Birthday Trust that persuaded the

Medical Research Council to conduct trials to show its safety for use by midwives. Trilene provided a much more portable, easily used form of analgesia which could be carried to the homes more readily than nitrous oxide. After the Second World War it was the Trust again that persuaded the Home Office to allow pethidine, the strongest analgesic used in childbirth by this time, to be used by midwives on their own; to this day the rules of pethidine usage by midwives acting independently are derived from the Trust's persuasion of the Home Office.

SURVEY WORK OF THE TRUST

As well as basic science and field research on analgesia, the National Birthday Trust pioneered many national surveys to examine the maternity services in the UK. In 1946 Professor J W B Douglas examined 14 000 births occurring in March of that year. This survey was conducted in conjunction with the Population Investigation Committee; results were published in *Maternity in Great Britain* (Douglas 1948). Information was collected on the effects of childbearing on the economics in the household; many medical aspects were not assessed but relief of pain in labour was analysed, and the methods of delivery were detailed.

In 1958 the National Birthday Trust combined with the Royal College of Obstetricians and Gynaecologists to sponsor a Perinatal Mortality Survey perfomed by Professors Neville Butler and Dennis Bonham. Here 17 000 births in one week in England, Wales and Scotland were surveyed using a detailed questionnaire completed by midwives at the time of delivery, examining antenatal and intrapartum care including use of pain relief. In addition, a subset analysis was performed for the subsequent 3 months of all stillbirths and neonatal first week deaths using extensive pathological facilities nationally to examine some 7 000 deaths. The results were reported in *Perinatal mortality* (Butler & Bonham 1963) and *Perinatal problems* (Butler & Alberman 1969) and have been used widely by administrators and doctors to plan some of the changes that occurred in the maternity services. Professor W C W Nixon, who had initiated the perinatal mortality survey, said:

> The perinatal death rate is also an index of the number of near deaths which may have occurred, [who] present with defects, acquired in pregnancy, at a later date. Like an iceberg, you see only a proportion of the end results, the deaths. But we must not forget the submerged and larger fraction, the near-deaths and the harm they will cause.
>
> The correlation is suggestive because some causes of death are known to be associated with occurrence of mental or physical defects in some of the survivors. With reduction in perinatal mortality there also follows pari passu, a diminution of perinatal morbidity.

Research is still being generated from these data. The whole concept of pregnancy among women of higher risk for maternal reasons took off from this study. Detailed analysis of these factors and a full account of the increased risks of maternal age and parity were investigated, as were the effects of cigarette smoking, shown here for the first time in a large national survey.

The next in the series was the British Survey 1970 by doctors Roma and Geoffrey Chamberlain under the joint auspices of the National Birthday Trust and the Royal College of Obstetricians and Gynaecologists. They investigated the care of the mother in pregnancy and labour (including analgesia). They examined particularly the first week after delivery and the quality of life of the child in that first week. They were purposely conscious of the live mother and baby, dealing with morbidity rather than mortality, for the previous survey had examined the latter. Again 17 000 births from England, Wales, Scotland and Northern Ireland were surveyed and the results were presented in *British births 1970*, volume 1 (Chamberlain et al 1975) and *British births 1970*, volume 2 (Chamberlain et al 1978):

From each of these first three surveys, cohorts of children were generated whose antenatal and intrapartum careers had been well documented. These were subject to further analysis and the children, now adults, are still being followed up by research teams such as those from the International Centre of Child Studies (in conjunction with the University of Bristol) and at the City University, London. More information is being extracted and published about the developmental and educational standards of the children who were born at the time of these studies and who have now become the parents of children of their own. This work will go on for many years; the first group of women are now approaching the menopause.

By the 1980s, the National Birthday Trust knew that other groups of doctors and social scientists in the Western world were becoming active in this field of data collection in relation to pregnancy and childbirth, following up the participants into subsequent life. The members of the Trust had also hoped at that time that the statutory collection of information was going to be expanded by the Government Statistical Service through the Offices of Populations, Censuses and Surveys (OPCS) so that much of the data which had been collected by the NBT surveys would then become available in Government statistics based on the information collected routinely from health professionals. Sadly this has not come about; the Statistical Services have been greatly reduced and there are large gaps in data collection and publication but the Trust did not know that in the mid-1980s. Demographic advice was that cohorts of children collected in the manner that the National Birthday Trust had used was not necessarily the best way of generating studies for long-term follow-up. The group of children might be biased in some way such as the type of women who filled in questionnaires or gave consent for their completion or by the season of the year in which the cohort of children were born; those might bias the population and influence educational and developmental factors. In consequence of these three trends the Trust decided not to perform further overall surveys of the whole maternity service but to concentrate on special aspects of the subject in future.

In 1984 the National Birthday Trust mounted a survey on the facilities available at the place of birth, giving the direction to Professor Geoffrey Chamberlain and Miss Phillipa Gunn, a midwife. The Survey would not be based upon individuals but would be place-orientated in England, Wales, Scotland and Northern Ireland, examining facilities available in hospitals, in GP units, or in the home where women were having babies. Questions were asked about staffing levels of midwives and doctors (obstetricians, anaesthetists and paediatricians) of all seniorities. Assessment was made of certain sample services such as blood transfusion, resuscitation equipment and dedicated operating theatres. The

plans and management structures laid down by the health authorities who ran the services were well known but the National Birthday Trust actually turned the stone over and looked at what was really being done. This survey assayed units, looking at staffing over 24 hours in samples over 4 months. The anaesthetic services were assessed, especially examining the availability of epidural anaesthetic which seemed to vary in close association with staffing levels.

The results were published in *Birthplace* (Chamberlain & Gunn 1987) and have been well received by the professionals in midwifery, obstetrics and anaesthetics and also by those planning maternity services into the more difficult years of the late 1980s and early 1990s. The advent of the new Health Service made *Birthplace* all the more valuable for it was the last national study before the greatest upheaval of the Health Service was thrust on to the unconsulted and surprised professionals.

THE PRESENT SURVEY

The National Birthday Trust decided to turn its attention to the current scene in pain relief in labour and members of the Trust wondered if what was really happening in the country could be assessed. There had been many local or regional studies about certain aspects of pain relief, but the Trust wanted to look at the problem as a whole subject in all its aspects. Pain is exceedingly difficult to measure for it is very much an individual thing; the assessment and quantification of perception are hard and it was realised from the beginning that this would be a difficult survey to mount. It was planned that the work should be a prospective study which would be descriptive; it must involve everybody who participated in the care of the labouring mother, including the woman herself and her partner in all places of confinement. The survey would look at the woman in labour from several different angles simultaneously. Opinions would be gathered from the woman herself, her partner, and the professionals who surrounded her – midwives mostly but also obstetricians, general practitioners and anaesthetists. Further, Trust members realised that, in an attitudinal subject like this, opinions change with time. What was perceived just after the event might not be the woman's attitudes later:

> When I first filled in the questionnaire, the pain was fresh in my mind and if you had given me this questionnaire then I would have said the pain was horrific. Now [6 weeks later] I'm not sure; as time goes on I am sure it will be the nicest experience I ever went through, with or without pain relief.

It is comments like this from mothers which make one realise that the collection of data on pain relief is very subjective and is affected by the reinforcement of subsequent events acting on the woman who actually had the pain and its management. Hence from the earliest stages, a two-stage enquiry was planned with an assessment made some weeks after the delivery.

In 1987 the National Birthday Trust set up a meeting of interested parties and from this a working party to advise on the planning of the enquiry. It was to be a meeting place of the professional bodies who had helped in the previous surveys and who it was hoped would be interested in examining pain relief in labour and women who had had babies. Professional organisations invited to this meeting included:

— Association of Anaesthetists
— British Medical Association
— British Paediatric Association
— Department of Health of England
— Department of Health and Social Services, Northern Ireland
— Faculty of Anaesthetists
— Faculty of Community Midwives
— Institute of Obstetrics and Gynaecology
— Medical Research Council
— National Birthday Trust Fund
— National Perinatal Epidemiology Unit
— Obstetrical Anaesthetists Association
— Office of Populations, Censuses and Surveys
— Population Investigation Committee
— Royal College of Midwives
— Royal College of Obstetricians and Gynaecologists
— Scottish Home and Health Department
— Welsh Office.

On this occasion, the National Birthday Trust considered it very important to have the help and cooperation from the women who went through labour and received pain relief and their partners. It was not practical to seek consultation of all mothers and so representatives were invited from the National Childbirth Trust and the Maternity Alliance.

The large working party was chaired by Professor Geoffrey Chamberlain; it met on several occasions discussing and assessing all the information which the various members felt would be needed to make a good survey from their own points of view. Over 8 months, information was sifted and the pragmatic probability of adequate data collection in a usable form was assessed. The questions were fined down and points were referred back to parent bodies. The Chairman met with the various groups individually and the National Birthday Trust was very grateful for all the time, thought and effort which members of those bodies gave at the crucial planning stage of the survey.

It was realised that with most surveys of this nature far too much information was collected and never analysed. Therefore the Working Party tried to see that any questions they asked had a reasonable chance of being answered in a precise and discriminatory way; if this was not so, they were not included. In their absence plenty of space was to be provided in the questionnaire for women to answer with their own comments in an unstructured fashion. The difficult decision was taken by the working group that the questionnaires would be offered to all women irrespective of outcome so that even those women who suffered a stillbirth, neonatal death or a baby with a congenital abnormality were asked to help by filling in a form. The response rate was obviously lower in this group but it led to some poignant but revealing comments:

> I have not been able to answer all your questions; our baby daughter died when she was 10 days old. We had complications with Caesarean section, she being 7 weeks premature weighing 5 lb 9 oz and healthy. She then caught a virus which led to renal failure, causing her death. I hope I have been some help with the survey.

Comments like this moved the survey team; they came to realise how important it was that women could express their views even at the sad times of high emotion such as this.

It was decided that this confidential enquiry should take place over one week in 1990 of all the places where women deliver. This would include the consultant-based hospital maternity units, combined consultant and general practitioner units, general practitioner units, home deliveries, independent, (private) and armed service hospitals. It was obvious that the only way to get at all of these would be through the midwives who are the constant attenders at deliveries and so the cooperation of the Royal College of Midwives and its representatives was sought and willingly given in this survey as in all previous National Birthday Trust studies.

The National Birthday Trust is grateful to the midwives all over the country who filled in the questionnaires and who catalysed the collection of data from all groups. We hoped that we might be able to collect data on about 13 000 deliveries during one week and this would give information about the availability of analgesia in all places where deliveries occurred. The Trust wished to examine the effectiveness of analgesia by comparing the assessment made by the women who received it, her partner, the midwife attending and relevant doctors such as obstetricians and anaesthetists who may have been there. The timing of pain relief was important and its relationship to what the woman expected from previous antenatal instruction was considered.

An especial aspect of this survey was the effort to find out more about the use and effectiveness of non-pharmacological methods of pain relief. Women using relaxation, breathing methods, TENS and hypnosis were especially assessed, for this is a growing area of interest and the Trust wished to put it in context with conventional medical analgesia.

> It is a pity hospitals do not do more to encourage women to have confidence in their own ability to get through their labour without the use of drugs.
>
> I think there is a difference between pain relief and coping with pain; relaxation and breathing is a good way of coping with pain, but not necessarily relieving it.

It was decided to attempt to look at the side-effects of analgesia both on the mother and the baby. It was realised it would be difficult but anaesthetic and paediatric colleagues have examined these problem.

SUPPORT

The survey was financed by the National Birthday Trust with the aid of a generous grant from the Department of Health for which the Trust is grateful. The initial planning was in the hands of the Working Party and the final preparations were supervised by the Scientific Committee of the National Birthday Trust. The tactics were worked out by Mrs Ann Wraight, the Midwife Coordinator appointed to the survey, and Professor Geoffrey Chamberlain. Mrs Sarah Reed was most helpful in the collection and computer analysis of data. She also coped happily with the numerous drafts of the report turning numerous amendments into tidy copy. The work was mostly done at St George's Hospital, London. The Trust is grateful to both the hospital authorities and to St George's Hospital Medical School for the space and the facilities that they offered for the running of this survey.

REFERENCES

Barnes J 1970 Happier birthdays. Midwives Chronicle 83: 406–11
Butler N, Alberman E 1969 Perinatal problems. E & S Livingstone, London
Butler N, Bonham D 1963 Perinatal mortality. E & S Livingstone, London

Chamberlain G, Gunn P 1987 Birthplace. Wright, Chichester
Chamberlain R, Chamberlain G, Howlett B, Claireaux A 1975 British births 1970. Volume 1: The first week of life. William Heinemann, London
Chamberlain G, Phillipp E, Harlett B, Masters K 1978 British births 1970. Volume 2: Obstetric care. William Heinemann, London
Douglas J 1948 Maternity in Great Britain. OUP, Oxford

3. Mounting the survey

A. Wraight

By the end of 1989, the Working Party had made its recommendations and the foundation of the survey had been laid. The building of the actual framework was organised by the Survey Coordinator, Ann Wraight, its Director, Professor Geoffrey Chamberlain, and by the Scientific Committee of the National Birthday Trust. Sarah Reed was appointed as Coordinator Assistant and Secretary to the project from April 1990. A timetable of the main events can be seen in Table 3.1.

IDENTIFICATION OF PLACES OF DELIVERY

All places of confinement within the UK were invited to participate in the study.

Our communication with the Directors of Midwifery Services (see Fig. 3.1) first began by contact with the Chief Nursing and Medical Officers in the Health Departments of the four countries, informing them of the proposed project. Once they had given their approval to the plan, we then wrote to the Regional Nursing Officers in England and their colleagues at the equivalent level in Scotland, Wales and Northern Ireland to inform them also of the study and to seek their agreement for their regions to take part. We requested from them the names and addresses of all NHS units providing maternity care within their authority and the appropriate persons with whom we should communicate. The majority gave the names of the Supervisors of Midwives or the Directors of Midwifery Services as we expected. Some, however, gave the names of the Director of Nursing Services or the Unit or District General Managers. To our dismay some weeks later, we discovered that agreement to participate

had been given by some of these non-midwifery senior managers without consultation with the Director of Midwifery Services.

The Ministry of Defence was contacted and once permission was granted all Army and RAF maternity units were invited to participate. The Royal Navy does not have an obstetric service in the UK, only overseas. The maternity units serving the Isle of Man and the Channel Islands and the independent hospitals were all approached separately.

The Supervisors of Midwives were asked to liaise with community and independent midwives so that women delivering at home could be included in the survey.

A willingness to participate was given by all senior administrative levels but when the request actually reached the Directors of Midwifery Services, 30 (9%) declined for the following reasons:

— Poor staffing levels
— Other surveys in progress
— High workload.

A further 7 units, who had agreed initially to take part, did not when the survey took place due to staff sickness and a greater than average delivery rate. This resulted in a total of 89% participation from all places of confinement in the UK (see Ch. 4).

ETHICS COMMITTEE APPROVAL

The previous maternity care evaluation surveys (1946, 1958, 1970 and 1984) had taken place before ethics committees were widely established. Since no National nor even Regional Ethics Committees existed, approval for the study had to be sought

17

Table 3.1 Timetable of the NBT 1990 Survey

	1989 Dec–Jan	1990 Feb–Mar	Apr–May	Jun–Jul	Aug–Sep	Oct–Nov	1991 Dec–Jan	Feb–Mar	Apr–May	Jun–Jul	Aug–Sep	Oct–Nov	1992 Dec–Jan	Feb–May
Advertising the survey		■	■											
Communicating with all involved	■	■	■	■										
Consulting with:														
Scientific Committee	■		■		■		■		■		■		■	
Statisticians	■	■				■	■				■			
NPEU[a] (Oxford)			■											
Developing questionnaire		■	■											
Pilot studies (2)			■											
Agreeing contracts:														
Printers			■											
Data entry firm			■											
Publishers								■						
Despatching questionnaire:														
Branches 1 and 2				■										
Branch 3					■									
Coding					■									
Data entering								■	■					
Editing						■	■	■						
Brainstorming							■							
Analysing										■	■	■		
Presenting findings												■	■	
Writing report													■	■

[a]National Perinatal Epidemiology Unit.

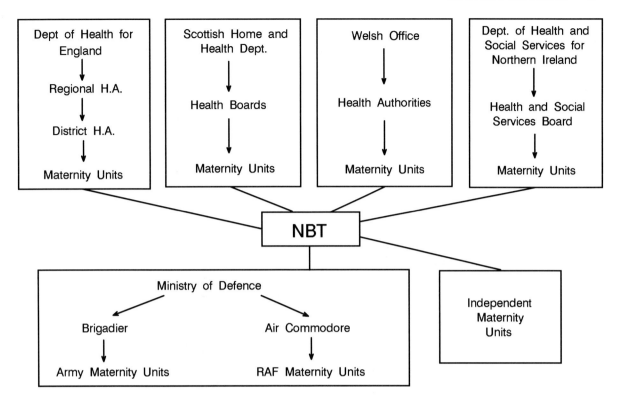

Fig. 3.1   Communications between the NBT team and the respondents.

from each District Ethics Committee independently. This was an enormous task but the majority of committees considered the study to be an audit of clinical care which did not involve any change or intrusion into treatment so they gave prompt and complete approval. Some requested more detailed information which involved answering complex questions, many of which were irrelevant to the purpose of the study. Some senior midwives asked the National Birthday Trust administrator to submit the forms for approval to ethics committees on their behalf. By the survey week, all 254 committees had given approval for the study to take place within their districts. This reflects a lot of extra work by the Survey Coordinator and her assistant and emphasises the need for a National Ethics Committee to guide local committees in their tasks when national surveys are planned.

RESEARCH METHODS

With such a large amount of data to collect from so many sites, the best research instrument was thought to be a postal questionnaire. This method has its advantages and disadvantages. Relatively lower cost is the major advantage over the telephone or face-to-face interview. No pressure is put on the respondent to give an immediate response so she can choose a convenient time to complete the questionnaire. Respondents have a greater feeling of anonymity and there is no risk of interview bias to influence the answers given. The major disadvantage is a reduced response, often less than 50% from target populations in the general public. The response rate is one of the main indices of data quality control in a survey because it defines the extent of possible bias from non-response. It is more difficult to create and maintain motivation in a written questionnaire, which can result in incompleteness and inaccuracies of responses to questions. Misunderstandings cannot be corrected nor questions answered as they can be in an interview. The survey is also completely reliant on an efficient postal service.

Data that were wanted to collect were accumulated by the members of the Working Party at committees; they were then edited and restructured with the help of members of the Scientific Committee of the National Birthday Trust and consultation with the statisticians and midwife researchers at the National Perinatal Epidemiology Unit in Oxford.

FEASIBILITY AND PILOT STUDIES

Once the questionnaires had been tested on a few independent women and midwives, we embarked on the first of two pilot studies.

In January 1990, in a pre-pilot survey, midwives at two local hospitals – St George's Hospital in London and Redhill Hospital in Surrey – were asked to complete questionnaires in each unit and to give comments about the structure of the questions and the notes of guidance. Their comments were valuable so the questionnaires were again edited and prepared for the pilot study.

In February 1990 six maternity units of varying size and location took part in the second pilot study which involved data collection from women having babies, their partners, their midwives and the doctors. We are grateful to the staff of and the women attending the following hospitals for accepting this double load: Daisy Hill Hospital, Newry, Northern Ireland; Furness General, Barrow in Furness, Cumbria; Humana Hospital, London; Morriston Hospital, Swansea, Wales; Princess of Wales RAF Hospital, Cambridgeshire; and St Helier Hospital, Carshalton, Surrey.

Data were collected on all deliveries within a 24-hour period in each unit; again comments made on the ease of completion and difficulties or misunderstandings were noted. The average time taken to complete Branch 2A, the professionals' part and omitting the first examination of the baby was 15 minutes, and so the survey team felt they had condensed the questionnaire down to an acceptable level. Data collection by this method must be pragmatic and we realised that even a quarter of an hour is a long time to give when it is at the end of a night shift and you want to get to bed.

PUBLICITY

While the planning of the study was in progress, the Director and Coordinator travelled to centres in the UK to publicise the survey. They spoke to audiences of midwives in England, Wales, Scotland and Northern Ireland, to obstetricians and obstetrical anaesthetists. The survey team also spoke to selected groups of women who were having or had just had babies. From all these groups, we learned of anxieties and areas which needed examination. Most were already in the survey but emphasis was changed after some discussion.

Information sheets were printed and sent to all interested consumer and professional organisations who wanted to be informed of the survey although they would not be taking an active part in the data collection. Descriptive articles were published in the medical, midwifery and national press describing the aims and process of the study. The Director described the aims and benefits of the proposed study in May 1990 on BBC Radio 4 and 5 in programmes to keep the women informed of the survey, our hope being they would participate if delivered in the relevant week.

THE QUESTIONNAIRE (SEE APPENDIX)

Information was collected in four questionnaires:

BRANCH 1. A senior midwife in each unit was asked to provide a profile of each maternity unit. This requested details of the type and size of unit, information on the previous year's work load such as babies under 2500 g and number of Caesarean sections. Simple measures of obstetric outcome such as perinatal mortality rates were also requested. We then enquired about analgesic methods available at the unit specifically asking for details about epidural anaesthesia. In this profile we assessed the availability of anaesthetists on the first day of the survey as a biopsy of the whole week.

BRANCH 2A. This was to be completed by the professionals involved. It included several parts, each to be completed separately by the midwives, obstetricians, general practitioners, anaesthetists, paediatricians or other professionals who examined the baby. Each part provided a profile of each woman, e.g. her age and parity; her labour and delivery, i.e. the onset and length of labour as well as the method of delivery; her pain control methods and their effectiveness as assessed by each professional involved in her care – this would include alternative methods and not just drugs; an assessment of the baby at delivery and at his first examination.

It would be necessary to include all these variables – independent, dependent and controlled – so that the response rates could be examined for bias, e.g. if more women from the upper social classes participated in this study. In addition in certain analyses, specific cases could be excluded to control the group, e.g. all multiparae could be excluded from the correlation of maternal age and method of pain relief used to produce a primiparous subset which provided more condensed data.

BRANCH 2B. This was to be completed by the woman and her partner or, in his absence, her supporter in labour. It provided information on the couple's preparation for labour and methods of analgesia planned comparing it with methods used. The woman's and the partner's assessment of the effectiveness of the methods were examined along with other factors which were helpful or unhelpful in pain relief. The initiation and choice of methods were both assessed, as was the analgesia used for perineal repair. Details of Caesarean section under general anaesthesia were requested and some idea of the effects of the analgesia on the woman and her baby was sought. In all, there were five lines of assessment for each method of pain relief used. The midwives, the obstetricians, the general practitioners, the anaesthetists, the women and the partners had the same rating scale so that the different assessments could be compared. Each respondent was asked to rate the method as 'very good', 'good', 'poor' or 'no use'. It will be noted that there is no midpoint category in this scale. This was done in an effort to force the respondent to rate in the extreme categories rather than in the middle, neutral category so as to avoid the bias towards a central tendency beloved of humans filling in questionnaires.

BRANCH 3. Six weeks after the main survey took place, further questionnaires were sent to a random sample of women who had expressed a willingness to participate in this follow-up survey. 1400 questionnaires were despatched to 25% of those who agreed to take part in this survey. This prospective study would provide details on the woman's perception of her care in labour and her pain relief as she assessed these now so that comparison could be made with her previous feelings expressed soon after the birth (see Ch. 10). Other details would include questions on her physical and emotional health, her relationship with her baby and the method of feeding. Reminder letters were sent to women who did not respond in this group but not to the respondents in the main survey.

CONFIDENTIALITY

Before the batches of questionnaires were sent out to the units, a unique survey number was given to each Branch 2A and 2B questionnaire. This number was recorded in the survey office in relation to the unit which received that questionnaire. On arrival back at the survey office, the same unit number was allocated to the Branch 1 forms as was used for Branch 2. In the returned questionnaires, all geographical details were removed so that the information was anonymous from now on. Hence only two people saw both the unit data and the survey number; such was the pressure of the numbers of forms being returned that no-one could possibly remember any links so that the survey was completely confidential.

Once the random sample had been done for Branch 3, the relevant survey numbers were copied and the personal details removed from Branch 2B. From this stage, all analysis was done on anonymous questionnaires, the different parts being linked by code numbers only.

To maintain confidentiality, no analyses were made at District Health Authority (DHA) level. In some DHAs all the deliveries would be grouped into a single hospital. Hence publication of DHA data could be equatable with single hospital information and the Trust felt this could breach confidentiality. By staying at regional level no specific maternity unit would be identified. The data from each unit would be grouped into Regions by which it would be analysed and reported. However, confidential information special to each maternity unit would be sent personally to the Head of Midwifery Services for her own and her staff's interest.

DESPATCHING OF THE QUESTIONNAIRES

The survey took place in the week commencing 25 June 1990 when data would be collected on all deliveries during that week. It was thought that a later date would have been inconvenient to the units as larger numbers of staff would be taking annual leave.

The approximate number of questionnaires required by each maternity unit had already been determined by requesting this information from the Directors of Midwifery Services. Errors occurred here both by underestimation (in most cases the rate was higher than average during that particular week of the survey) or overestimation when the monthly rate was given by mistake resulting in four times the number of questionnaires needed being despatched.

The actual packaging and posting of the questionnaires was a slow and time-consuming exercise. Records were made of the destination of all the questionnaires before they were packaged and then each parcel had to be weighed independently and stamped accordingly. Delays in the printing of the questionnaires meant that a very short period of time was left for their preparation and despatch.

By 15 June 1990, 504 parcels of varying size and weight comprising a total of 14 504 questionnaires had been posted to the units. The cost was £1225 and business reply labels were enclosed to cover the return postage. This involved volunteer help in transportation and postal formalities. The Trust is grateful to Patrick Wraight for his willing participation and time given in this task.

During the weeks of the survey, several units requested more questionnaires and some photocopied extra copies to cope with the larger than average birth rate on that week. Some had difficulty in completing a questionnaire for every birth because the week was such a busy one. It was later estimated that during that particular week the birth rate was over 15 000 – an increase of 2000 over the estimated weekly average.

THE RETURNS

The first questionnaire was returned on the second day of the survey, 26 June 1990, the last reaching our office on 19 March 1991 – 37 weeks after the survey had ended. A small but appropriate floral reward was sent to the coordinator of the first unit.

The final figures for the study are shown in Table 3.2.

DATA PREPARATION AND ANALYSIS

The survey office was at St George's Hospital Medical School where both statistical and computing services were available. The keying-in of the data was done by an external company experienced in the handling of large data sets. The data cleaning, merging of the data sets and data analysis were all done on computers at St George's Hospital linked to the Amdahl at the University of London Computer Centre (ULCC) using the MVS service with the Phoenix command language and the Statistical Analysis System (SAS) software. This work was done by survey staff but they were greatly helped by Dr Valerie Dickinson and Mr Richard Hulkhory from the computing department at St George's Hospital. The analysis was done under the guidance of the statistical department led by Dr Martin Bland, Senior Lecturer at St George's Hospital Medical School. We are especially grateful to two statisticians, Ashley Pottier and Janet Peacock, who acted both as teachers and troubleshooters through the whole process of editing and analysis from December 1990 to September 1991.

The processing of the data was not without its problems, mainly due to the size of the study. Most of the answers in the questionnaires had been precoded which resulted in a considerable saving of time. A few answers, however, were not capable of such sophistication but it had been realised from the planning stage that an open-ended response would be the only valid one in such an attitudinal study. We planned as few as possible of these; an average of 10 minutes was required to check each form and code the open-ended areas numerically. Poorly completed forms were discarded at this stage.

Table 3.2 The questionnaires returned and the response rates (NBT Survey 1990)

Questionnaires	Potential response	Actual response	Response Rate (%)
Branch 1. Profile of unit	330	293	(89)
Branch 2a. Professionals	c.15 000	10 352	(66)
Branch 2b. Consumers	c.15 000	6459	(41)
Branch 3. Follow-up	1400	1149	(82)

The first batch of coded forms was despatched for punching in August 1990 and all the punching was completed in February 1991. This lengthy period of time resulted from major errors being discovered at the first analysis stage so that tapes and even questionnaires on one occasion had to be returned for re-keying.

Editing of the material commenced as soon as the first tapes arrived at the survey office. Data from the tapes were copied onto disk and filed in the form of SAS data libraries at the University of London Computer Centre. Frequency distribution tables of every variable on each questionnaire were produced and examined for obvious errors, e.g. a baby's weight of 8 kg, a woman's age of 63 years. Since these were not keying errors but occurred at the time of completion of the questionnaire, the appropriate maternity units had to be contacted to clarify the problems.

Once all the data had been cleaned, the disks were merged so that cross tabulations could be done between the variables in all sections of the study. The SAS system was chosen because of its ability to merge, sort, update and manipulate large data collections of different lengths and totals. The mainframe computer at the University of London Computer Centre was capable of handling a data set of this size – a valuable asset. The majority of the analysis was done on this system, but some analysis on specific variables only was done on a personal computer by downloading the relevant data onto a separate disk. The choice of analysis method was made by the individual author. Professor Philip Steer particularly chose this method (see Chs 5 and 6) as he was already expert at analysis on his own computer. Tests of statistical significance (i.e. t-test and chi-squared) were used where relevant to establish whether differences between groups were likely to be real or whether they had occurred by chance.

BRAINSTORMING

Once the data had been cleaned and the initial analyses were being sorted, it was thought wise to reconsult with midwives, obstetricians and National Childbirth Trust teachers – to identify their particular needs from the data that were known to be available. Each group brought different suggestions suited to its particular outlook and extra analyses were done to provide the information. The survey team found this exercise to be very helpful and have included many of the suggestions and requests in this report but in some cases requests exceeded the data we held so that the survey could not be used to answer the questions.

REPORT OF FINDINGS

The mounting of this study was complex because it involved the collation of data from different people – professionals and consumers. The responsibility for this lay on the shoulders of the midwives who not only had to complete their section of the questionnaire but also had to encourage the other staff involved with that delivery as well as the woman herself and her partner to complete their parts. The National Birthday Trust appreciates the extra work that this entailed for midwives already stretched to their limits on busy delivery suites and is very grateful to those who responded so well and so enthusiastically. Because the midwives had the greatest involvement in the study the Director considered that the first report on the preliminary findings should be to the midwives themselves. This presentation took place at an enthusiastic meeting of the Heads of Midwifery Services in October 1991, which was attended by some 200 midwives, members of the National Birthday Trust and the Presidents of both the Royal College of Midwives and the National Birthday Trust. The National Birthday Trust is grateful to the Royal College of Midwives for hosting that event.

Brief oral reports were given in 1992 to representative groups of senior and research orientated midwives and by invitation to obstetricians at the 26th Congress of Obstetrics and Gynaecology at Manchester.

CONCLUSIONS

The Pain Relief in Childbirth survey was a descriptive, prospective study involving everyone who participates in the care of labouring women including the women themselves in all places of confinement within the UK. Those involved believe that the measurement of pain in labour, albeit difficult, and its relief by analgesics or alternative methods, are central to care. As a leading article in the *Lancet* in 1953 commented:

> If our aim is to do the best we can for the mother we must take all her needs into account, neither exposing her to wasteful needless pain, nor depriving her too officiously from control of her great occasion.

The study provides a description of the methods in use in 1990 and their effectiveness assessed by the woman, her partner and her professional supporters.

4. The hospitals and the women who used them

G. Chamberlain

In the last week of June 1990, most women having babies in the UK delivered in hospitals. Of these, 10 353 women had data in the National Birthday Trust survey; 48 did not deliver in hospital, of whom 32 of these were delivered at home with booked planned confinement, the others delivering either unexpectedly at home or in transport between the home and the hospital. These women are considered in Chapter 8. The remaining 99.5% of women delivered in a hospital and are considered in this chapter.

TYPE OF UNIT

When planning the survey, we approached Regional and District midwifery offices and, with their agreement, we wrote to their nominated representatives in all the hospitals listed in the *NHS Hospital Year Book for England, Wales, Scotland and Northern Ireland 1989*, and to yet others that the Supervisors of Midwives told us about. Details are shown in Table 4.1 to compare with the units which took part in a similar analysis done by the Trust 6 years before. Three-quarters of women delivered in National Health Service hospitals run

by consultants with or without GP facilities; some 20% delivered in isolated GP units. These ranged from moderately large cottage hospitals to small units doing one delivery a week only. The remaining 5% delivered in Armed Services hospitals or in the private sector. Figure 4.1 shows that in comparison with the survey of only 6 years before, there has been a great shutdown in all units performing obstetric care from 531 to 293, a reduction of 238 units or 44.8%. Some 141 of these came from the isolated GP sector and 94 from the consultant NHS units.

Table 4.2 is condensed from 4.1 and shows the groupings of hospitals indicating an increase in 16.5% of NHS consultant units, with a concomitant decrease of 17.7% of isolated GP units.

SIZE OF UNIT

The trend in the National Health Service is to close smaller, isolated units. They are hard to staff at a standard expected in 1990. The numbers of doctors and midwives are limited and appropriate equipment needed for emergencies is expensive. This is one of the problems which society must address. Many women and some professionals prefer the pleasantness of the small unit with its more personal touch; others use the argument that small units are less economic to run than larger ones. Putting financial considerations apart, it is certainly more difficult to maintain facilities in the smaller units which lack the critical size required by medical Royal Colleges and faculties for recognition of junior medical training posts. One is reminded of Aneurin Bevan's comment in the debate setting up the National Health Service in 1946:

Table 4.1 The types of units (NBT Survey 1984 and 1990)

	1984 n	1984 (%)	1990 n	1990 (%)
NHS consultant unit	195	(36.7)	132	(45)
NHS consultant and GP unit	114	(21.5)	84	(28.6)
NHS consultant and private unit	9	(1.1)	6	(2.1)
Isolated GP unit	199	(37.5)	58	(19.8)
Armed Services	6	(1.1)	4	(1.4)
Private	6	(1.1)	6	(2.1)
Other	2	(0.4)	2	(0.7)
Not known	0	(0)	1	(0.3)
TOTAL	531	(99.4)	293	(100.0)

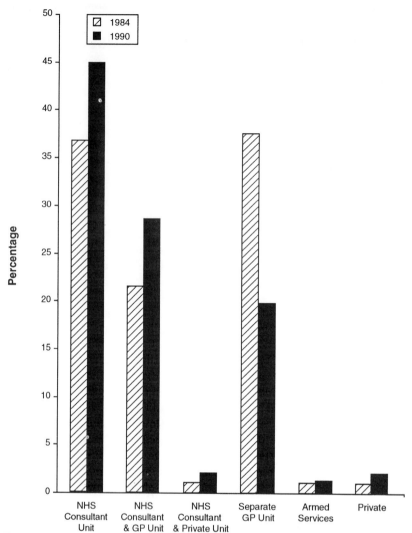

Fig. 4.1   Types of units in the NBT Surveys 1984 and 1990.

I would rather be kept alive in the efficient, if cold, altruism of a large hospital than expire in a gush of warm sympathy in a small one. (Foot 1973)

Table 4.2   Condensed data by rates from Table 4.1 (NBT Surveys 1984 and 1990)

	1984 %	1990 %	Change %
NHS consultant units	59.3	75.8	+ 16.5
Isolated GP units	37.5	19.8	− 17.7
Other units	2.3	5.2	+ 2.9

It is perhaps not the economics that should be guiding us but the capacity to provide safe facilities for mothers and babies which will cause this trend to continue.

In the 1984 survey, we divided units up by their size; this seemed a helpful device. Table 4.3 indicates their distribution in 1990, and Figure 4.2 compares these data with those of 1984.

A *small unit* is one where less than 500 women a year gave birth; whilst a quarter of the units in the country were in this size group they only account for 2% of deliveries. These are mostly isolated GP units.

A *medium unit* is one where between 501 and 2000 women a year delivered; another quarter fall

Table 4.3 Units by size and number of deliveries (NBT Survey 1990)

Size (deliveries per year)	n	Units (%)	Deliveries	Total deliveries (%)
Small (1–500)	67	(23)	242	(2)
Medium (501–2000)	72	(25)	1921	(15)
Large (2001–4000)	118	(40)	6960	(56)
Very large (over 4000)	35	(12)	3344	(27)
TOTAL	292	(100)	12467	(100)

into this group, and they delivered only 15% of the population in the year before the survey. Hence about half of the units of the country performed only 17% of the deliveries in 1990.

A *large unit* is one where between 2001 and 4000 women a year gave birth. These make up 40% of the units and are mostly District General Hospitals. 56% of deliveries took place in these units, the majority of women.

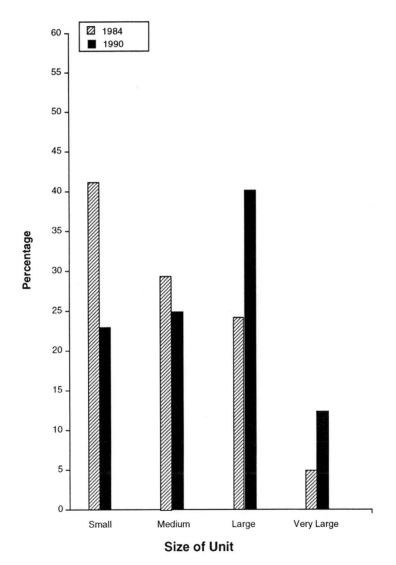

Fig. 4.2 Percentage of units in the NBT surveys, 1984 and 1990
Small – up to 500 deliveries per year.
Medium – 501–1999 deliveries per year.
Large – 2001–3999 deliveries per year.
Very large – 4000 or more deliveries per year.

A *very large unit* is one where more than 4000 women a year gave birth, the largest being over 6000 deliveries a year. They only constitute 12% of the units, but because of their size they deliver about a quarter of the women. Hence in 1990 it can be seen that 83% of women deliver in units that perform over 2000 deliveries a year. This helps to allow adequate staffing rates and expertise to provide the services the women expect.

The trend of the move to the larger unit is shown again in Table 4.4 and Figure 4.3. In the 6 years since the last survey, the number of medium and small units was reduced from 68.8% to 48%. Probably more significantly, they now look after only 17% of deliveries, compared with 33% previ-

Table 4.4 Comparison of rates of size of units and number of deliveries (NBT Surveys 1984 and 1990)

	1984		1990	
Size of unit	Units (%)	Deliveries (%)	Units (%)	Deliveries (%)
Small	40.8	5	23	2
Medium	28.0	28	25	15
Large	24.2	50	40	56
Very Large	4.9	17	12	27

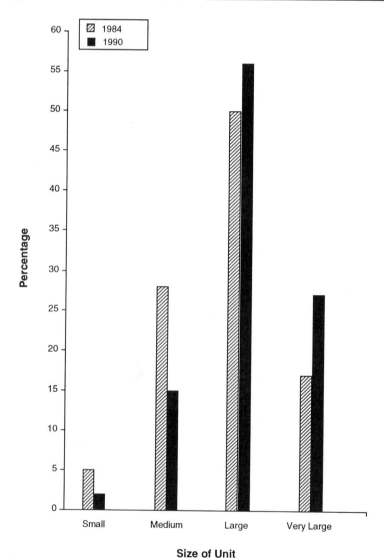

Fig. 4.3 Percentage of deliveries in different sized units (NBT 1984, 1990) size of units as outlined in Fig. 4.2.

ously. The number of births in the larger units has increased proportionally; whereas they looked after 67% in 1984, 83% of the women now deliver there.

WORK LOAD

When further analysis of the units and the number of deliveries they performed was done by regions, a wide diversity was seen. As might be expected, with its ranging geography, Scotland has many more small units whilst more urban areas like South West Thames and Mersey have none.

The use made of these units is shown in Table 4.5. For example, there were 64 deliveries in the survey week reported from 26 small units in Scotland, that is 2.5 deliveries per unit. This compares with the rather brisker throughput of the West Midlands where 44 deliveries took place in 5 small units (8.8 deliveries per unit). Similar ratios can be derived in the other size units but, perhaps because of the larger figures involved in analyses, they seem to even off in the very large units where 80 to 120 deliveries a week have been reported.

Figure 4.4 shows the percentage of women in each Region who deliver in units reporting over

2000 births per year. Another measure of the workload in a unit could be derived by examining a sample of a work intensive mechanism; Caesarean sections are easy to identify and utilise many doctors, midwives and others in the unit in much extra work. Table 4.6 shows the units by the number of Caesarean sections performed in the previous year. A constant association between the size of the unit and the number of Caesarean sections done can be seen going regularly across the table.

PERINATAL MORTALITY RATE

In 1989 the perinatal mortality rate (PNMR) in England, Wales, Scotland and Northern Ireland was

Table 4.6 Number of Caesarean sections (CS) in previous year by size of unit (NBT Survey 1990)

Size of unit	CS reported in year				TOTAL
	<50	51–200	201–500	>500	
Small	65	2	0	0	67
Medium	6	46	20	0	72
Large	1	1	103	13	118
Very large	1	0	5	29	35
TOTAL	73	49	128	42	292

Table 4.5 Units and deliveries by region (NBT Survey 1990)

Region	Small Units n	Small Del. n	Medium Units n	Medium Del. n	Large Units n	Large Del. n	Very large Units n	Very large Del. n	Totals Units n	Totals Del. n
Northern	1	4	9	259	2	72	1	63	13	398
Yorkshire	1	7	5	178	9	422	2	182	17	789
Trent	1	7	3	83	7	377	5	556	16	1023
East Anglia	2	8	1	13	6	312	2	156	11	489
North West Thames	0	0	2	50	10	524	2	179	14	753
North East Thames	3	21	2	43	14	906	0	0	19	970
South East Thames	1	0	2	39	10	623	0	0	10	662
South West Thames	0	0	3	99	9	485	1	80	13	664
Wessex	1	0	2	78	4	262	1	129	8	469
Oxford	0	0	0	0	4	251	3	333	7	584
South Western	5	15	1	32	5	302	3	279	14	628
West Midlands	5	44	2	27	10	597	6	549	23	1217
Mersey	0	0	2	60	3	190	2	176	7	426
North Western	5	15	4	113	7	468	4	385	20	981
Channel Islands	0	0	2	38	0	0	0	0	2	38
Northern Ireland	0	0	10	212	4	303	0	0	14	515
Scotland	26	64	11	364	9	499	2	212	48	1139
Wales	10	19	7	169	7	367	1	65	25	620
Armed Services	1	9	3	36	0	0	0	0	4	45
Independent	5	29	1	28	0	0	0	0	6	57
TOTAL	67	242	72	1921	120	6960	35	3344	291	12 467

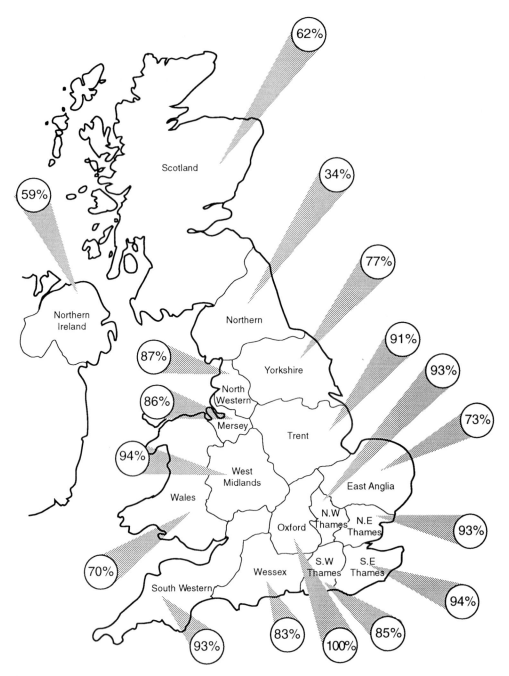

Fig. 4.4   Percentage of women in each Region who deliver in units reporting over 2000 births per year (NBT 1990).

approximately 9 per 1000 total births. All the units had been asked to give their perinatal mortality rate for that year or the previous year of 1988. The number of units in each Region that had a PNMR

below 9 per 1000 and those with a perinatal mortality rate of and above 9 per 1000 are shown in Table 4.7 and Figure 4.5. The southern Regions reported that over 60% of their units had a PNMR below 9 per 1000, one Region having twelve out of thirteen units in this group. The smallest proportions of units with a PNMR below 9 per 1000 were found in the North Western Region, West Midlands, Northern Ireland and Wales. These Regions are often associated with problems of congenital abnormalities and low birth weight. The data on the proportion of units with PNMR of 9 per 1000 and above are less firm. The North Western Region is the only one where there were more units with a PNMR of 9 per 1000 and above than those reporting a lower level, although Northern Ireland came close to this. The problem of missing data on perinatal mortality will be discussed later and it makes these data unreliable for statistical evaluation. However, there is a trend seen here which fits with other nationally derived data.

A similar analysis was made of the proportions of units in each Region that reported deliveries of low birth weight babies (under 2500 g) in the previous year. This is a mixed measure of outcome involving both the background population and the obstetrical services provided. Results are shown in Table 4.8 and Figure 4.6, but are not so revealing as are the data on PNMR, possibly because of this compendium of factors. The highest rate of units reporting

Table 4.8 The numbers and proportion of units reporting low birth weight babies (under 2500 g) classified by Region (NBT Survey 1990)

Region	Total units	Units delivering more than 200 babies annually with a birth weight <2500 g	
	n	n	(%)
Northern	13	1	(8)
Yorkshire	17	5	(29)
Trent	16	8	(50)
East Anglia	11	2	(18)
North West Thames	14	6	(43)
North East Thames	19	4	(21)
South East Thames	10	4	(40)
South West Thames	13	3	(23)
Wessex	8	1	(13)
Oxford	7	3	(43)
South Western	14	3	(21)
West Midlands	23	7	(30)
Mersey	7	1	(14)
North Western	20	4	(20)
Channel Islands	2	0	(0)
Northern Ireland	14	1	(7)
Scotland	48	4	(8)
Wales	25	2	(8)
Armed Services	4	0	(0)
Independent	6	0	(0)
TOTAL	291	59	

Table 4.7 Perinatal mortality rates per 1000 total births in recent year reported by units (excluding in utero transfers) divided at a rate of 8.99/1000 (NBT Survey 1990; see text for unused data comment)

Region	Total units n	PNMR < 9 n	(%)	PNMR ≥ 9 n	(%)	No Data n	(%)
Northern	13	7	(54)	2	(15)	4	(31)
Yorkshire	17	9	(53)	2	(12)	6	(35)
Trent	16	9	(56)	2	(13)	5	(31)
East Anglia	11	8	(73)	0	(0)	3	(27)
North West Thames	14	8	(62)	0	(0)	6	(38)
North East Thames	19	16	(84)	0	(0)	3	(16)
South East Thames	10	8	(80)	2	(20)	0	(0)
South West Thames	13	12	(93)	1	(7)	0	(0)
Wessex	8	5	(63)	1	(13)	2	(24)
Oxford	7	6	(86)	1	(14)	0	(0)
South Western	14	7	(50)	0	(0)	7	(50)
West Midlands	23	10	(43)	7	(30)	6	(27)
Mersey	7	5	(71)	0	(0)	2	(29)
North Western	20	4	(20)	8	(40)	8	(40)
Channel Islands	2	2	(100)	0	(0)	0	(0)
Northern Ireland	14	6	(43)	5	(36)	3	(21)
Scotland	48	28	(58)	5	(10)	16	(32)
Wales	25	10	(40)	7	(28)	7	(32)
Armed Services	4	4	(100)	0	(0)	0	(0)
Independent	6	4	(67)	0	(0)	2	(33)
TOTAL	291	168		43		80	

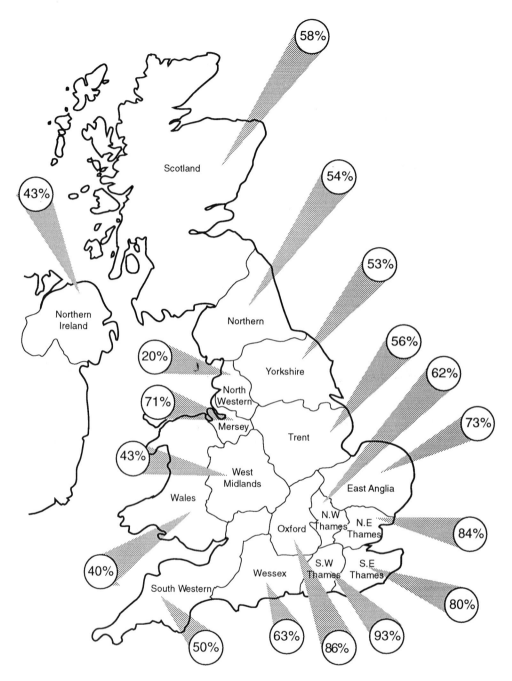

Fig. 4.5 Percentage of units in each Region reporting a perinatal mortality rate of less than 9 per 1000 total births in the year 1989 (NBT 1990).

low birth weight are in Trent, where half the units had delivered more than 200 low birth weight babies the previous year. Similarly, higher proportions were noted in North West and South East Thames and in the Oxfordshire Region. Those Regions with a higher proportion should have been linked with a higher PNMR but North Western, West Midlands and Northern Ireland did not report

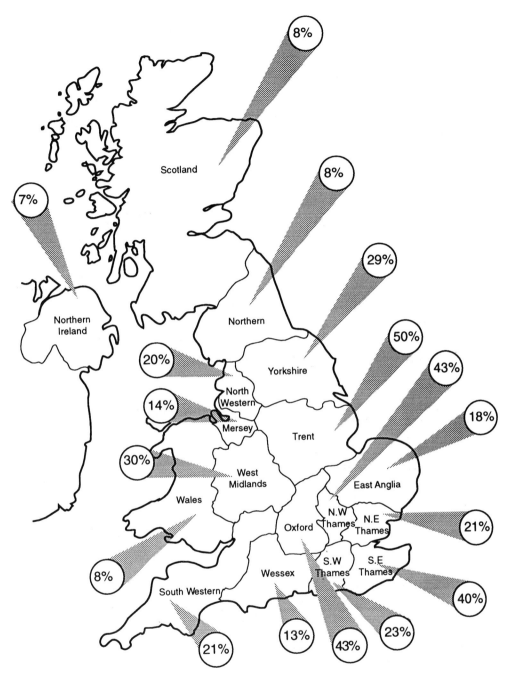

Fig. 4.6 Percentage of units in each Region reporting more than 200 low birth weight babies (less than 2500 g) born in the previous year (NBT 1990).

a particularly high proportion of units with low birth weights. This may be because these Regions have a higher use of in utero transfers, and so concentrate their deliveries of low birth weight babies in a smaller number of units with neonatal intensive care facilities. Thus the degree of the problem would not show on this simple unit derived analysis.

MISSING UNITS AND DATA

Among the hospitals in the country, 37 could not participate in this survey. A further 4 did not complete Branch 1 but did participate in other parts of the survey and so analyses of Branches 2a, 2b and 3 include these units. In the past the National Birthday Trust has relied upon the participation of the midwives and other hospital staff to fill in forms; response rates of over 90% of hospitals have always been achieved in the previous surveys (see Table 4.9 and Fig. 4.7). On this occasion it was only 89%. We understand the extra load that has been put onto the midwifery service, and that there are more questionnaires arriving in the post each week. At the time of our survey, the regrading of midwives was fresh in the mind and causing much controversy. The reorganisation of the Health Service was rumbling on the horizon and many midwifery and hospital managers felt hard pressed. A further small, but worrying cause for concern for future surveys, is that now a certain number of survey organisers are offering financial inducements for completing the forms. A charity organisation like the National Birthday Trust could never compete on these grounds. For example, at the rate of an inducement of £5 per form filled in, it would cost more for inducements than for all the expenses of the rest of the 1990 survey put together.

These are reasons for non-compliance rather than excuses. The small non-cooperation rate was uniform throughout the UK. It would be invidious to list those units that could not help; probably those who work in and manage these units will still make use of and benefit from the results of this survey performed with other people's efforts, though having not contributed themselves.

The units that did not participate included four small ones, three medium, three large and four very large hospitals. While the first two groups would make very little difference, the latter two

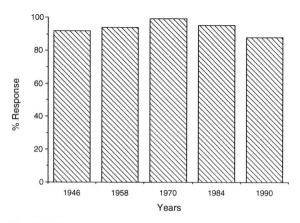

Fig. 4.7   The percentage of units responding to the National Birthday Trust studies in the last 45 years.
1946 Maternity in Britain
1958 Perinatal Mortality
1970 British Births
1984 Place of Birth
1990 Pain in Labour

could mean a loss of up to 600 deliveries in the week compared with the 10 000 approximately that we did collect information on. Hence, although we lost 12% of units, we missed 6% of women delivering at them – in addition to those who, although delivering at participating units, did not return their forms.

Of those units which did participate, a certain number could not give us data on their background information for the previous year under certain headings. These are shown in Table 4.10. Whilst it is understandable that statistics on items like in utero transfers would be difficult to extract, the perinatal mortality rate and low birth weight information should have been well known inside any unit. With the new Health Service organisation and the advent of medical audit in obstetrics, comparisons are supposed to be made between the past and the present, hoping to show improvements. How can we do this in the midwifery service when 56 out of 293 units could not give even a perinatal mortality rate for a recent year?

THE WOMEN

When a survey looks at a sample of the total, it must be careful that the sample is representative. We therefore examined our sample of 10 185 women by

Table 4.9   Percentage response of units and women to the five NBT Surveys

Year	Units (%)	Women delivered (%)
1946	92	91
1958	94	98
1970	99	98
1984	95	99
1990	89	66

Table 4.10 Data not obtained from participating hospitals in Branch 1 (NBT Survey 1990)

Region	Low birth weight	In utero transfers	Perinatal mortality rate	Anaesthetic cover
Northern	1	3	3	—
Yorkshire	2	5	3	1
Trent	1	4	4	1
East Anglia	1	1	—	—
North West Thames	2	3	2	—
North East Thames	2	6	2	—
South East Thames	—	4	4	—
South West Thames	—	—	—	1
Wessex	—	1	—	—
Oxford	—	1	—	—
South Western	—	1	4	1
West Midlands	4	3	1	6
Mersey	—	1	1	—
North Western	2	5	6	6
Channel Islands	—	—	—	—
Northern Ireland	—	3	3	—
Scotland	—	4	13	11
Wales	2	1	9	6
Armed Services	—	2	—	—
Independent	—	2	1	—

various social and biological factors to see how they fitted with the total population. At the time of writing this analysis, national data for 1990 were not available for England and Wales or Northern Ireland, and so we had to use the data of 1989, which is probably close enough. In addition, in changing from Hospital Inpatient Enquiry to Korner Core data sets, much information was not collected so that even the 1989–90 maternity data are incomplete and are based on only 55% of the expected number of maternity episodes. We used data of England and Wales, which represented some 90% of the women who would have been in the population. The Scottish data, although available, was in a slightly different form, and this was considered to make comparisons difficult. We feel that these two minor differences in time and population will not cause major bias.

Age

Table 4.11 and Figure 4.8 show data on maternal age. A concomitance is seen between the women of the National Birthday Trust survey and the total population. There is a slight shift in the survey group from the 35–39-year age group into the 30–34, but this is small.

Table 4.11 Age of mothers delivering (NBT Survey 1990 and 1989 England and Wales population; see text)

Age	NBT Survey		1989 E & W	
	n	(%)	n	(%)
≤ 19	722	(8.1)	55 522	(8.1)
20–24	2 348	(26.4)	184 414	(27.0)
25–29	3 121	(35.2)	241 018	(35.3)
30–34	1 984	(22.3)	143 794	(21.1)
35–39	592	(6.7)	48 944	(7.2)
≥ 40	112	(1.3)	9 387	(1.3)
TOTAL	8 879	(100.0)	683 079	(100.0)

Parity

In the survey group there were 42.2% nulliparae and 57.8% multiparae. There was a slight increase in the proportions of multigravidae among the black and Asian populations (61.8% and 63.5% respectively), but otherwise the proportions were similar to the national figures of 39.9% nulliparae and 60.1% multiparae.

Social class

Socioeconomic classification was derived from the occupation of the partner or husband; if he was unemployed this was recorded as a separate category (Table 4.12 and Fig. 4.9). As always a large

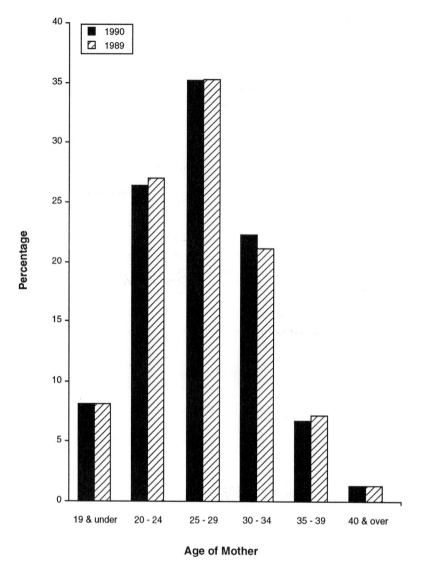

Fig. 4.8 Percentage of women delivering by age group in the NBT Survey 1990 and 1989 total population – see text.

number were unclassifiable and a certain number were not known. Generally, 17.1% of the survey group were in social classes I and II and 16.9% were social classes IV and V. This is a distinct and significant difference from national data on England and Wales, where 25.2% are in social classes I and II and 12.9% social classes IV and V. Further, the unclassifiable and unclassified groups were of a lower proportion in the survey. As a result of this shift, we had many more social class III (non-

manual and manual) in our survey than in the general population (41.0% cf. 31.8%).

Country of origin

The midwife was asked the country of origin of the mother and given the choice shown in the questionnaire (see Appendix, Branch 2A). This resulted in the data shown in Table 4.13; the vast majority were white (92.0%), which compared with 91.6% in

Table 4.12   Socioeconomic class of partner (NBT Survey 1990 and 1989 England and Wales population; see text)

Class	1990			1989		
	n	%		*n* 1000s	%	
I	583	5.7	} 17.6	194.2	25.2	
II	1 209	11.9				
III non-manual	1 500	14.7	} 41.0	57.6	7.3	} 31.8
III manual	2 676	26.3		226.0	24.5	
IV	1 363	13.4	} 16.9	128.4	12.9	
V	356	3.5				
Unemployed	869	8.5	} 24.5			
Unclassifiable	1 420	13.9		48.7	30.1	
Not Known	209	2.1				
TOTAL	10 185	100		654.9	100	

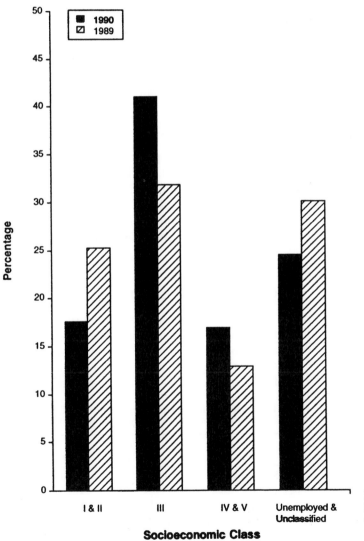

Fig. 4.9   The percentage of women delivering by socioeconomic class in the NBT Survey 1990 and the 1989 total population – see text.

Table 4.13 Country of origin of the mother (NBT 1990 and 1989 England and Wales population; see text)

Ethnic origin	n	Survey %	1989 %
White	9 372	92.0	91.2
Carribbean	107	1.0	0.6
African	72	0.7 } 1.0	1.7
Other black	33	0.3	
Indian	189	1.9	1.3
Pakistan	156	1.5	1.8
Bangladesh	36	0.4	0.7
Chinese	37	0.4 } 1.3	0.8
Other Asian	93	0.9	
Other	97	1.0	1.9
Not known	161	1.6	0
TOTAL (known)	10 192	100	100

the England and Wales population. The black group in this survey was 2.0% compared with 2.3%; the others were of such small proportions that the minor variations between the survey and the general population are not significant. The apparent discrepancy in the proportion of blacks reported in this survey was probably because the black women when asked in this survey considered themselves to be British. They were neither African nor Caribbean for they themselves had been born in this country. This represents one of the common problems in collecting data on racial origin.

We asked in the survey about interpreters, their need and their use. Table 4.14 shows that very few were needed, but where they were required they were mostly available, particularly for the Asian and black populations.

Marriage and support

The marital status and support of the mother are shown in Table 4.15. 71.5% of survey responders were married compared with 73.8% of England and Wales population. Of the remainder, the distribution between single, separated, divorced and widowed is approximately the same as in previous

Table 4.14 The requirements, usage and availability of an interpreter (NBT Survey 1990)

	White	Black	Asian	Other
Interpreter deemed necessary	26	5	115	21
Interpreter used in labour	5	4	89	19
Availability	19%	80%	77%	90%

Table 4.15 Status and support of mothers (NBT Survey 1990)

Marital status	n	(%)
Married	7247	(71.5)
Single	2517	(24.8)
Separated	151	(1.5)
Divorced	215	(2.1)
Widowed	8	(0.1)
TOTAL	10 138	(100)

Support	n	(%)
Supported	9678	(95.7)
Unsupported	432	(4.3)
TOTAL	10 110	(100)

surveys although there were no data available for England and Wales for 1989 at the time we analysed the survey. A second question was asked about the degree of support, for although 28.8% were single many of these were in a stable union. The data of the survey responders showed that 95.7% of all women (that is married and unmarried) considered themselves to be supported and only 4.3% in the survey group were unsupported.

Multiple pregnancies

Data about multiple pregnancies in the survey are reported in Table 4.16. There were 103 sets of twins and 1 set of triplets. National data show these to be within the expected range allowing for small figure variation. With our small numbers, we could show no variation amongst mothers from different countries of origin.

OBSTETRICAL FEATURES

The National Birthday Trust 1990 survey differed from that of 1984 because information was collected about individual women. This in no way was intended to provide material to start a cohort analysis for long-term follow-up, but was essential to assess

Table 4.16 Multiple pregnancies reported (NBT Survey 1990 and 1989 England and Wales population; see text)

	1990 n	(%)	1989 n	(%)
Singletons	9949	(99.1)	675 155	(98.9)
Twins	103	91.0)	7579	(1.5)
Triplets	1	(0.01)	183	(0.03)
Quadruplets or more	0	(0)	12	(0)

the perceived needs and efficacy of the pain relief methods in different obstetrical circumstances. In consequence, a picture is derived about a sample of 10 185 women who had questionnaires filled in by midwives, as occurred in previous surveys. Not all questionnaires were completed for each question but the data sheets contain enough information to give a picture of obstetrics in 1990 in the UK.

The obstetric history

This was assessed in the Branch 2B questionnaire from answers about the numbers of previous live births, stillbirths, abortions (early pregnancy losses) and neonatal deaths. From this can be derived certain characteristics. The perinatal mortality rate in previous deliveries for the 6240 multiparous women in the survey was 12.1 per 1000 total births. This would fit with the perinatal mortality rates of the years immediately before the survey was performed. The past early pregnancy loss rate was 23.7%. There are no national data available on abortion rates but our data fit into the range expected of reported miscarriages.

Antenatal problems occurring in pregnancy (Table 4.17)

By far the commonest problem in the current pregnancy was hypertension; the question does not differentiate between that associated with pregnancy and that induced by the pregnancy. These data would fit approximately with other currently reported surveys of hypertension. Antepartum haemorrhage data are not collected nationally. The last National Birthday Trust survey to collect individual data was in 1970; this reported a total vaginal bleeding rate of 10.5% in pregnancy, of which 4.7% was before 28 weeks, thus about 5% of women bled in the last 28 weeks of pregnancy. This is consid-

Table 4.17 Some reported antenatal problems of 10 182 women (NBT Survey 1990)

Antenatal problem	n
Raised blood pressure	843
Antepartum haemorrhage	210
Intrauterine growth retardation	311
Prolonged rupture of membranes	274
Cardiac disease	77

erably greater than the proportion reported in this survey, but the two data sets perhaps do not allow one to compare like with like.

Intrauterine growth retardation and premature rupture of membranes are reported in approximately the same rates as in other published surveys. The data on cardiac illness are not recorded nationally; these consisted very much of what was perceived to be a cardiac illness by the mother so it varied from coarctation of the aorta down to physiological vascular murmurs which are clinically not significant.

Length of pregnancy

Data were collected and grouped as shown in Table 4.18 and Figure 4.10. Information on gestational age is not usually published nationally; we have compared the 1990 National Birthday Trust survey data with the last NBT survey of 1970 where individual data were collected. It will be seen that there is a shift between the two surveys so that many more women delivered between 37 and 40 weeks. This is almost entirely at the expense of the 41+ weeks group. This may not be a real effect, because in 1990 ultrasound dating of pregnancies had become almost universal whereas in 1970 its availability was very limited. Thus many women delivering at what they thought was 43 weeks in 1970 were probably earlier in gestation than they imagined (30% of women are certain of the date of their last menstrual period when they book). The same caveat will apply to some of the preterm births.

Induction and augmentation of labour

Since this survey was not specifically about labour but about pain relief during labour, the questions on

Table 4.18 Gestational age of singletons at delivery (NBT Surveys 1970 and 1990)

Gestational age	1990 n	(%)	1970 n	(%)[a]
<24 weeks	3	(0)	0	(0)
24–28 weeks	27	(0.3)	99	(0.6)
29–32 weeks	91	(0.9)	163	(1.0)
33–36 weeks	426	(4.3)	776	(4.9)
37–40 weeks	7055	(70.4)	9587	(60.1)
41–42 weeks	2407	(24.0)	4603	(28.8)
≥43 weeks	14	(0.1)	739	(4.6)
Not known	677		858	

[a]Of those known.

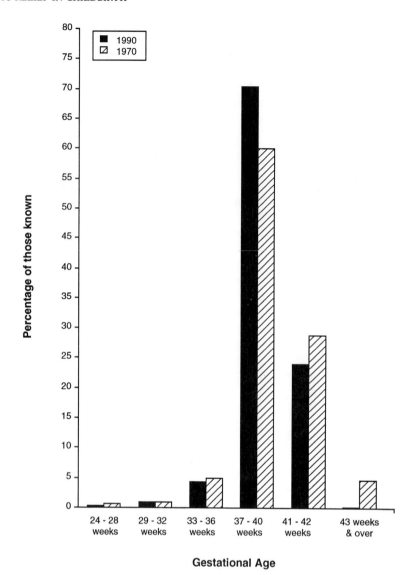

Fig. 4.10   Percentage of women by gestational age at delivery in NBT 1970 and 1990 Surveys – see text.

induction or augmentation were put together. It was the effect of the method of induction or augmentation that was needed and so these figures should not be taken as those on induction alone. In many cases either Syntocinon or artificial rupture of the membranes were performed once labour had started naturally.

The data are given on Table 4.19 where the three major methods of induction and augmentation are considered. The figures for prostaglandins are probably those of induction only for there are no grounds currently for using prostaglandins once labour has really started; they represent 14.2% of the population who entered data on this subject. Among these, 40% received prostaglandins alone and the rest of women had other methods in addition. This probably is not the true figure of prostaglandins alone for the use of artificial rupture of the membranes or Syntocinon may have come later in the labour, not truly at induction. It is still a surprisingly small number of women who are not being given this efficient method of induction.

Table 4.19 Induction and augmentation (NBT Survey 1990; see text)

Induction and augmentation	n	%[a]	%[b]	%[c]
ARM alone	1609	51.1		
+ Syntocinon	851	27.0		
+ prostaglandins	334	10.6		
+ Syntocinon and prostaglandins	356	11.3		
All ARM	3150		32.1	66.3
Syntocinon alone	903	40.5		
+ ARM	851	37.9		
+ prostaglandins	134	6.0		
+ ARM and prostaglandins	356	15.9		
All Syntocinon	2244		22.2	47.2
Prostaglandins alone	563	40.6		
+ ARM	334	24.1		
+ Syntocinon	134	9.7		
+ ARM and Syntocinon	356	25.7		
All prostaglandins	1387		14.2	29.2

[a]Percentage in induced groups.
[b]Percentage of total population (n = 9763).
[c]Percentage of those induced (n = 4750).

Syntocinon was used alone for 903 women, and alone or in combination with ARM and/or prostaglandins for about one-fifth of the population (2244 women). Artificial rupture of membranes, which may have been in labour or to start labour, was used in two-thirds of women, being used alone in just over half.

The reasons for an induction were specifically asked for; amongst those who responded to this question 11.3% were induced and this may be nearer to the real percentage of inductions as opposed to augmentations.

Table 4.20 lists the principal reasons given, of which prolonged pregnancy and raised blood pressure are the major two single reasons. The others are as might be expected. From this table it would seem that 11.3% of women were induced. This might be an underrepresentation, for induction rates in the United Kingdom are reported to be

Table 4.20 Indications for induction (NBT Survey 1990)

Indication	n	(%)
Prolonged pregnancy	485	(41.6)
Raised blood pressure	210	(18.0)
Prolonged rupture of membranes	146	(12.5)
Fetal health	92	(7.9)
IUGR	75	(6.4)
Poor past obstetric history	32	(2.6)
Other recorded indication	127	(11.0)
TOTAL	1167	(100.0)

between 15 and 25% of total populations (18% from the Maternity Hospital Episode Statistics 1989–90 (Department of Health 1991)). This range is wide because with the cuts in the governmental statistical branch there have been no really reliable national data on this since 1987. Some idea of this problem of underrepresentation is given by the fact that only 92 women out of over 10 000 had an induction for poor fetal health, which would include abnormalities in fetal heart rate pattern, although some women with fetal indications may be hidden in the other groups, e.g. those induced on the indication of raised blood pressure or prolonged pregnancy.

Method of delivery

The method of delivery was given in all but 264 reports and the details are shown in Table 4.21 and Figure 4.11.

Some 79% of women had a spontaneous vaginal delivery, 10% had an operative vaginal delivery with forceps or vacuum extraction, and 11.4% a Caesarean section. These figures approximate to those in the national data; we have difficulty in getting the precise figures of operative deliveries and Caesarean section rates from England and Wales because the Department of Health changed the data collection systems in the late 1980s. They

Table 4.21 Method of delivery (NBT Survey 1990 and 1989 England and Wales population)

Method of delivery		1990	1989
	n	(%)	(%)
Spontaneous			
OA	7622	(75.5)	
OP	219	(2.2)	
Breech	76	(0.8)	
Face	21	(0.2)	
TOTAL		(78.7)	(78)
Vaginal instrument			
Forceps	736	(7.3)	
Vacuum extraction	190	(1.9)	
Breech	74	(0.7)	
TOTAL		(9.9)	(9)
Caesarean section			
Before labour			
Elective	470	(4.7)	
Emergency	125	(1.2)	
In labour	556	(5.5)	
TOTAL		(11.4)	(11)
Not known	264	(2.5)	(2)

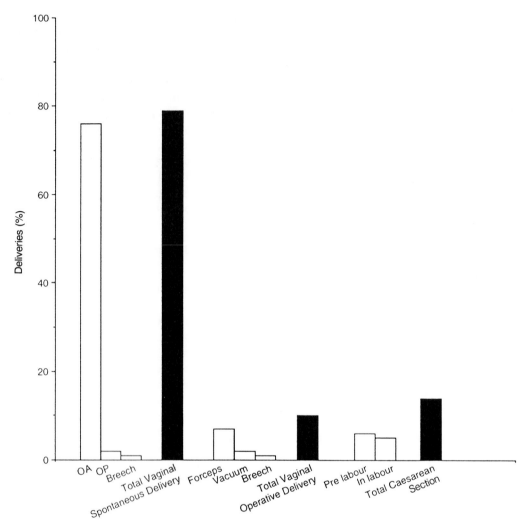

Fig. 4.11   Percentage of deliveries by various methods. The black bars indicate the total spontaneous vaginal deliveries, total operative vaginal deliveries and total Caesarean sections (NBT 1990).

gave up one system before implementing another, so that there is a gap of some years and one can only make generalisations about operative delivery rates at the moment. Based on a 55% sample the Department of Health can say that in England and Wales in the financial year 1989–90, instrumental vaginal deliveries make up 9% and Caesarean sections 12%. These are in the same zone as the National Birthday Trust survey.

Birth weight

The birth weight was recorded in all but 760

instances. Table 4.22 and Figure 4.12 compare the birth weights of the survey babies with those born in the national cohort in 1989. Unfortunately the national cohort stops detailed recording at 3500 g and groups all the larger babies together, and again the data are also not broken down for those under 1500 g. Although the numbers less than 1500 g are small, they are an important group and we understand that OPCS are taking steps to change the classifications of published data soon. Comparison shows that the survey is underrepresented in the smaller babies; in the under 2500 g birth weight group, the survey only included 5.5% of babies

Table 4.22 Birth weights of babies (NBT Survey 1990 and 1989 England and Wales population)

Birth weight (g)	1990 n	(%)	1989 n	(%)
<1500	74	(0.8)	7388	(1.1)
1500–1999	80	(0.8)	9288	(1.3)
2000–2499	377	(3.9)	30 167	(4.3)
2500–2999	1537	(16.0)	145 738	(20.8)
3000–3499	3550	(37.0)	249 795	(35.7)
3500–3999	2893	(30.2)		
4000–4499	922	(9.6) (41.5)	257 511	(36.8)
4500–4999	134	(1.4)		
≥5000	26	(0.3)		
Not known	760			
TOTAL	10 353	100	699 887	(100)

whereas the national data contain 6.7%. Similarly only 16% of survey babies were in the 2500–3000 g birth weight group whereas 21% of the national cohort were in this group. This bias is confirmed by the overreporting of those over 3500 g. It would seem therefore that the survey has a bias towards women who had babies with a heavier birth weight answering the questionnaires.

CONCLUSIONS

Despite its size the survey is not completely representative of the population of England and Wales. Because of the non-participation of certain hospitals

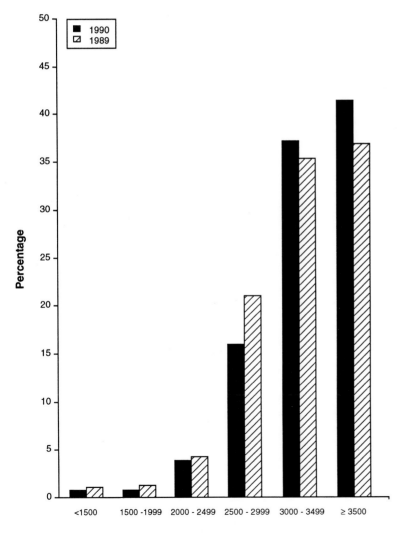

Fig. 4.12 The percentage of babies by birth weights in the NBT Survey 1990 and the 1989 total population – see text.

and the patchy returns of those participating in the survey, more data are missing than in previous National Birthday Trust surveys. The data missing may well include the more problematic cases and so the survey is left illustrating the groups at the better end of the spectrum. For example, the birth-weight changes and the methods of delivery would indicate a bias towards the better endowed obstetrically. It is always this group which is prepared to fill in questionnaires and take the trouble to give a half hour of their time when there are many other distractions calling upon them. In a survey of this nature, another confounding variable is that those who have something to say will fill in the questionnaires, hence one might expect the two ends of the opinion spectrum to be over-represented compared with the large silent majority who were basically satisfied with what they had.

REFERENCES

Department of Health 1991 Maternity hospital episode statistics 1989–90. HMSO, London
Foot M 1973 Aneurin Bevan. Paladin, St Albans, Herts, vol 2 p 131

5. The availability of pain relief

P. Steer

THE ORIGIN OF PAIN IN LABOUR

> I think the most important thing about pain relief is to have all options open and to be able to select the right one for you at the time.

The experience of pain in labour is presumably as old as the human race (see Ch. 1). It is not only the contractions of the uterus per se which are painful, but the dilatation of the cervix which accompanies them during labour. The human uterus is spontaneously contractile, and isolated human muscle suspended in a nutrient, oxygenated solution contracts every 3–4 minutes without external stimulus. In early pregnancy, the massive amounts of progesterone produced initially by the corpus luteum of the ovaries and then subsequently by the placenta serve to suppress obvious uterine contractions until about 24 weeks gestation, when contractions begin to be noticed. These contractions, called Braxton Hicks contractions after a nineteenth century London obstetrician, are relatively painless because there is no accompanying dilatation of the cervix. An important signal that pregnancy is changing into labour is the beginning of pain with each contraction. Thus a common definition of the onset of labour is 'the occurrence of regular *painful* contractions every 5–10 minutes'. Other signs that labour is imminent are the passage of a show (a slightly blood-stained plug of the mucus that normally seals the cervix during pregnancy against the ingress of bacteria) or spontaneous rupture of the amniotic membranes. Both of these events are usually secondary to the widening of the cervical orifice.

The functional value of pain due to dilatation of the cervix is not known for sure, but it can be conjectured that it is a signal to the mother that the important event of birth is about to take place. Unexpected delivery in an unsuitable environment is a hazard even under the optimum conditions of modern civilised society, and presumably was at least as dangerous under the harsher conditions prevailing in prehistoric society. Thus the pain of labour may be imagined as a signal to the expectant mother to find a suitable safe haven (secure from animal attack, warm and draught free) before the birth of the child.

If the function of pain in labour is to provide a warning, and this warning is heeded, then one may hypothesise that there is no need for the pain to continue. If this hypothesis is true then pain may be relieved without any inevitable adverse effect on the mother, fetus, or progress of labour. In other contexts, the relief of pain is seen as appropriate once the function of the pain has been completed. For example, the pain of a hot flame on the skin of the finger prompts removal of the hand from danger. Inappropriate pain relief would increase damage by allowing the person to stay in their damaging situation. However, once away from the flame, the pain of a burn can safely be removed by appropriate means, and it would be considered inhumane not to do so.

METHODS OF PAIN RELIEF IN LABOUR

The argument over whether relief of pain in labour is appropriate has centred around the discussion of whether the pain has anything other than a warning function. Theologists attempted to prevent early use of agents such as chloroform for pain relief in labour with the argument that the Bible stated 'in sorrow thou shalt bring forth children' (Genesis 3:16), the pain being a punishment for Eve's temptation of Adam; thus, relieving pain was frustrating the will of God. Queen Victoria, who first used chloroform in 1853 when in labour with the eighth of her many children, was said to be most impressed with its effects and this largely quelled opposition in polite society to the use of analgesia in labour.

There can be no doubt that in childbirth, as in other aspects of life, psychological state and preparation have a major influence upon the way events are experienced. Personality also has a powerful effect; all accoucheurs are familiar with the scenario of the apparently calm and well prepared mother who goes to pieces during labour, while an anxious hypochondriac may cope surprisingly well. It seems likely that almost any psychological technique can help ameliorate pain in labour, provided the woman also has knowledge, confidence and support. Probably the only psychological technique which can remove pain entirely is hypnosis but only about 25% of women are suitable deep trance hypnotic subjects. In addition, to be effective, the technique relies on extensive preparation, often taking 20 or more hours of face to face contact with the hypnotist, and the attendance of the hypnotist is also required throughout most of labour. The same is true of acupuncture. On the other hand, side-effects are rare.

Transcutaneous electrical nerve stimulation (TENS) employs the gate principle of pain control, so that the sending of impulses in one set of nerves competitively blocks the perception of impulses from another set of nerves. The technique produces feelings of pins and needles in the back and legs, blocking the nerves carrying pain signals from the cervix. TENS probably works best with chronic low level pain, and thus is reasonably effective in early labour; however, such trials as have been performed do not suggest a statistically significant benefit in advanced labour (Harrison et al 1986).

The most widely used analgesic currently is pethidine (meperidine or Demerol in the US). It was discovered during a search for new muscle relaxants and developed as an analgesic in Germany during the early 1940s to replace morphine. It stimulates receptors in the brain normally activated by endorphins, *endo*genous mor*phine*-like substances, which are produced naturally in response to acute pain. Pethidine deadens pain rather than relieving it entirely, and its effect varies from person to person. In some it causes euphoria while in others it causes nausea and vomiting. It is often associated with drowsiness so that women may apparently fall asleep between contractions; this drowsiness may be manifested in the newborn as respiratory depression and this is the major disadvantage of the drug. It is, however, much better in this respect than morphine, as far less crosses the placenta and even less crosses the fetal blood–brain barrier. In addition, the synthetic opiate antagonist naloxone, when injected intramuscularly into the newborn infant, reverses the effects of pethidine within several minutes. Midwives in the UK are empowered to administer up to 150 mg of pethidine in labour on two occasions, without requiring a specific prescription from a medical practitioner.

Midwives are also able to administer freely nitrous oxide and oxygen gases (usually in 50% mixtures) for short-term pain relief. The commercially available premixed gas mixture, Entonox, is given from a pressurised storage cylinder through a reduction valve and is inhaled by the mother through a face mask. It is a weak anaesthetic and has only a short-term effect once inhalation stops. Women are therefore usually recommended to begin inhaling it at the beginning of a contraction, and stop once the peak of the contraction has passed. As with pethidine, its effect is somewhat unpredictable and ranges from good to negligible. It has almost no side-effects and, being very short acting, does not produce respiratory depression in the newborn infant.

The only current technique able to produce complete pain relief in a woman regardless of her personality type is epidural anaesthesia. The technique consists of injecting solutions of local anaesthetic into the epidural space between the lining of the body canal of the spine and the membranes covering the nerves from the spinal cord. The relatively long-acting agent bupivacaine is used widely, while lignocaine is sometimes used for rapid short-term effect. The drug is injected intermittently, or sometimes infused continuously through a narrow plastic catheter inserted into the epidural space by an anaesthetist. 85% of women who use it obtain total or almost total pain relief, while only 3% have no worthwhile analgesia.

Complications are unfortunately more common with epidural anaesthesia than with the methods previously described. The major problem is that the ability to move the legs is often lost along with the pain, effectively confining the woman to bed, in the lateral recumbent or sitting position; the supine position should be avoided because of the significant risk of a serious fall in blood pressure due to compression of the inferior vena cava, the largest vein draining blood from the lower half of the body. Some women find the feeling of numbness in the lower half of the body unpleasant, although in most cases they feel this is a small price to pay for the relief of pain. A drop in blood pressure occurs in about 15% of women, causing temporary reduction of blood flow to the placenta, following the first injection of local anaesthetic. This can be reduced to 5% if preloading with a litre of crystalloid solution such as Hartmann's solution infused intravenously in the 5 or 10 minutes prior to the initial dose.

Puncture of the dural membranes can occur – a dural tap – allowing leakage of cerebrospinal fluid. Because of the relatively large diameter of the needle used to allow passage of the plastic epidural catheter, a dural tap can result in the loss of a significant amount of fluid, which then causes a severe headache over the next 48 hours. The woman should be nursed flat during this time, and sometimes a blood patch is produced by an injection of the mother's own blood into the site so that a clot forms, blocking the hole. The incidence of this relatively uncommon complication depends substantially upon the skill and experience of the anaesthetist, but, even in a service with a high proportion of learners, should not exceed 1%.

Because of the loss of motor power in the abdominal muscles, and the reduced impetus from no longer feeling the urge to bear down in the second stage, the proportion of nulliparous mothers requiring forceps delivery or vacuum extraction is approximately doubled with epidural anaesthesia.

Recent reports have suggested a significant increase in long-term backache following epidural anaesthesia. This does not occur if the epidural is given for elective Caesarean section, suggesting that it is awkward movements while anaesthetised which may be to blame (MacArthur et al 1992).

Very rarely the injection of local anaesthetic enters the spinal fluid, causing ascending paralysis with eventual cessation of breathing so that the mother has to be intubated and ventilated until the anaesthetic wears off. For this reason, epidurals should only be used in maternity units which have full anaesthetic cover with experienced anaesthetists on 24-hour call, proper facilities for cardiopulmonary resuscitation and long-term ventilation if required.

METHODS OF PAIN RELIEF AVAILABLE IN THE UK IN 1990

Approximately 15 900 women gave birth in the UK in the study week. Of these, at least one part of the questionnaire was returned in 10 702 cases. 293 obstetric units participated in the study.

The availability of analgesic drugs was reported by 288 units. The most ubiquitous was Entonox, which was available in 99% of units (285), followed closely by pethidine, available in 97.6% (281). Epidural anaesthesia was only available in 73.3% of units (211). Other drugs available in a few units included morphine, diamorphine (or heroin), Omnopon, meptazinol (Meptid), pentazocine (Fortral), and midazolam (Hypnovel). The combinations of the drugs most commonly used are shown in Table 5.1.

When epidurals were provided, they were available on request at any time in 163 units (77.2% of those providing epidurals). They were available on request from 09.00–17.00h Monday to Friday in a further 13 units (6.2%). In 20 units (9.5%) they

Table 5.1 The availability of drugs for pain relief (NBT Survey 1990)

	Number of units	(%)
Entonox, pethidine and epidural	151	(52.4)
Entonox and pethidine	60	(20.8)
Entonox, pethidine, epidural and other	56	(19.4)
Entonox, pethidine and other	13	(4.5)
Entonox, epidural and other	3	(1)
Entonox only	2	(0.7)
Epidural only	1	(0.3)
Pethidine only	1	(0.3)
Other only	1	(0.3)

were available at any time but only for medical indications. In the final 15 (7.1%) they were available from 09.00–17.00h Monday to Friday for medical indications only.

> Personally I cannot understand why women need to go through the stages of pain that in other fields of medicine would be considered unacceptable. Surely if an epidural or some other form of effective pain relief is available it should be administered when requested. (partner's comment)

269 units said they offered or supported non-pharmacological methods of pain relief. 246 (91.5%) said they supported relaxation, and 174 (64.7%) TENS. Hypnosis and acupuncture were each available in 19. The various combinations offered or supported are shown in Table 5.2.

> Although she was in great pain some of the time, the fact that she was not drugged in any way meant that we could communicate and respond to each other very quickly. That is why the relaxation worked because I could verbally encourage her to relax. (partner's comment)

Table 5.2 The availability of non-drug methods for pain relief (NBT Survey 1990)

Method	Number of units	%
TENS and relaxation	146	(54.3)
Relaxation alone	71	(26.4)
TENS alone	18	(6.7)
TENS, relaxation and hypnosis	12	(4.5)
TENS, relaxation and acupuncture	10	(3.7)
Acupuncture alone	3	(1.1)
All the above	3	(1.1)
Acupuncture and relaxation	2	(0.7)
Hypnosis and relaxation	2	(0.7)
Acupuncture and hypnosis	1	(0.4)
Hypnosis alone	1	(0.4)

292 units (99.6%) indicated the professional who advised the woman about the methods of pain relief she might choose. The sources of advice involved the midwife in 284 units (97.2%), the obstetrician in 166 units (56.8%) and the anaesthetist in 117 units (40%). In 13 units the decision was also influenced by the GP or physiotherapist, with student midwives, homeopathists and acupuncturists also being mentioned in a few cases. These figures are summarised in Table 5.3.

> Good advice helps and our midwife was able to counsel very helpfully with relaxation techniques and with two drugs. I am certain the constant presence of a midwife in early, middle and late labour is crucial. (partner's comment)
>
> The staff had a difficult time in advising without leading. They were determined to let Mum make up her own mind (Dad on side lines) to the extent that they were at risk of getting no decision made at all or a late decision. Advice should be tendered without fear or favour. If Mum does not know how can she choose the most appropriate? (partner's comment)

Table 5.3 The professionals who advise women about pain relief (NBT Survey 1990)

	Number of units	(%)
Midwife	93	(32.2)
Midwife, obstetrician and anaesthetist	92	(31.5)
Midwife and obstetrician	57	(19.5)
Midwife and anaesthetist	18	(6.2)
Midwife and other	13	(4.5)
Midwife, obstetrician and other	6	(2)
Midwife, obstetrician, anaesthetist and other	5	(1.7)
Obstetrician only	4	(1.4)
Obstetrician and anaesthetist	2	(0.7)
Other	1	(0.3)

REFERENCES

Harrison R F, Woods T, Shore M, Mathews G, Unwin A 1986 Pain relief in labour using transcutaneous electrical nerve stimulation (TENS). British Journal of Obstetrics and Gynaecology 93: 739–746

MacArthur C, Lewis M, Knox E C 1992 Longterm problems after epidural anaesthesia. British Medical Journal 304: 1279–1282

6. The methods of pain relief used

P. Steer

Deciding what women actually used was made more complicated by the fact that only 6459 women completed their part of the questionnaire and, of these, only 6093 recorded the method of pain relief they used. In addition, the methods recorded by the women and the attending midwives differed in a large number of cases. The left-hand column of Table 6.1 lists the number of women recording the various methods of analgesia, arranged in descending order as a percentage of 6093. The middle column lists the corresponding frequency as recorded by the midwives, as a percentage of 10 352. The right-hand column lists the number of times the woman's record was corroborated by the midwife, and then expresses this as a percentage of the woman's total.

Of the four most popular methods, the percentage usage recorded by the woman and the midwife is the same within 2.2% in three. In these cases, the proportion of women whose choice is corroborated by the midwife is very similar, between 74% and

79.4%. Thus it seems likely that in just over 20% of cases where the woman's questionnaire has been completed, the midwife has just failed to complete her section.

Thus it can be stated with some confidence that approximately 60% of women used Entonox, 37% pethidine, and 18% epidural anaesthesia. It is interesting to note that 34% of women considered that they used relaxation as a method of analgesia, compared with only 3.8% of midwives who recorded it as a method used. Either midwives failed to notice that relaxation was being used, or they considered it was not a true method of analgesia. A similar recording deficit is noted in relation to massage, which women rated fifth in usage (19%) compared with only 4.8% of midwives who considered it worth recording.

It is curious that both women and midwives recorded general anaesthesia (GA) as a form of pain relief in a significant but different number of cases (3.9% and 0.8%). While medical staff usually regard

Table 6.1 The frequency of analgesic methods used as recorded by the women, their midwives, or both (NBT Survey 1990; see text)

Method	Women		Midwives		Both	
	n	(%)	*n*	(%)	*n*	(%)
Entonox	3665	(60.0)	5706	(55.1)	2700	(74.0)
Pethidine	2247	(36.9)	3918	(37.8)	1783	(79.4)
Relaxation	2073	(34.0)	406	(3.9)	143	(6.9)
Epidural	1178	(19.3)	1834	(17.7)	872	(74.0)
Massage	1178	(19.3)	515	(5.0)	174	(14.7)
TENS	335	(5.5)	428	(4.1)	235	(70.0)
GA	238	(3.9)	82	(0.79)	17	(7.1)
Diamorphine	128	(2.1)	375	(3.6)	83	(65.0)
Meptazinol	107	(1.8)	337	(3.3)	80	(75.0)
Homeopathy	22	(0.4)	21	(0.2)	5	(23.0)
Hypnosis	4	(0.07)	1	(0.01)	1	(25.0)
Acupuncture	1	(0.02)	2	(0.02)	1	(50.0)
TOTAL	6093		10 352		6093	

general anaesthesia as an adjunct to operative therapy, they often fail to realise that in offering a relief from pain it may also be seen as a method of analgesia by women. However, like relaxation, the perception of general anaesthesia as a method of pain relief is much more common amongst the women themselves than among the professional staff, a folk memory of the days of chloroform and ether in childbirth.

Although there is a perception that TENS is a popular method, due to its high profile in the media of recent years, in fact it was only the seventh most common in actual use. Only 5.5% of women on their own record used it at any time during labour.

Unlike the methods so far mentioned, diamorphine and meptazinol were less often mentioned by the woman than by the midwife. This is probably because they are less familiar to the general public than the more common methods. Although meptazinol has been promoted as an analgesic in labour for about twenty years, it is surprising that diamorphine (heroin) is still so widely used in view of its association with drug addiction and the administrative problems of it still being kept on the labour ward.

Despite their high profile in the media, the use of homeopathy, hypnosis and acupuncture is used by a small minority only, comprising less than 1% of analgesia used even when added together (see Table 6.1).

> Hypnotherapy is a specialised form of pain relief only applicable to people who have deep beliefs in it and are susceptible to hypnosis. When it works with the right person, as in my wife, it is extremely effective and when working properly no other pain relief is required – strength of mind is enough if sufficient belief is present.

When considering the overall choice of analgesia, it must be borne in mind that choice will be limited by the local availability of the various methods. For example, if only units where an epidural service was available on demand 24 hours a day 7 days a week were considered, and elective Caesarean sections were excluded, the rate of epidural usage (midwives questionnaire) was 24.4% (2041/8363). The use of

pethidine in women not choosing an epidural amounted to another 32.3% (2701/8363), 22.3% used other pharmacological methods (1870/8363) and only 20.9% (1750/8863) used no drugs at any time.

In the analysis which follows, because of the tendency of midwives to ignore methods such as relaxation and massage, the women's own questionnaires have been used as the base for analysis of the various factors influencing choice. This also gives added consistency when the woman's responses are compared with her planned form of analgesia, her predicted choice of analgesia in the next pregnancy, and for those who answered the follow-up form at 6 weeks.

In addition, the data set was selected to consider only women ticking at least one option relating to pain relief on the questionnaire, on the basis that women not ticking any alternative (including none, relaxation and breathing and massage as well as the pharmacological methods) had failed to cooperate. This conclusion appears justified as most of them also failed to check any of the options on the rest of the form. Women using only other methods were also excluded as the numbers were too small to analyse. Together these procedures removed 224 cases.

A further 434 women failed to record their planned method of analgesia, and an additional 313 declined to suggest a preferred method in a future pregnancy. They were also excluded from the subset analysis (see below).

Women having a planned Caesarean section (468) were then also excluded, as it seemed unreasonable to consider their analgesia in labour when they had no labour.

Women with a multiple pregnancy or breech presentation were also not considered, because their experience of labour is not typical and because their choice of analgesia is likely to be heavily constrained and taken on medical advice. This excluded a further 138.

These standardisations left a final data subset containing the responses of 4516 women who had experienced labour with a single fetus in cephalic presentation and who had completed their options for planned, used and future analgesia. This data set was used for the analyses which follow.

FREQUENCY OF USE OF THE VARIOUS METHODS IN INDIVIDUAL UNITS

Questionnaires of women who fitted the subset criteria were returned from 282 units. The mean number of questionnaires returned from each unit was 22, with a mode of 10. The minimum was one and the maximum 87. The distribution was strongly skewed, as shown in Figure 6.1.

In 116 units (41%) no-one completed labour without analgesia. In 223 units (79%) less than 10% of women completed labour without analgesia. The distribution of the percentages of women completing labour without pain relief is shown in Figure 6.2.

The use of massage was also uncommon; in 76 units (26%) no-one used massage for pain relief in labour. The distribution is shown in Figure 6.3.

Of the technological methods, TENS was the least common. In 160 units (57%) no-one used it in the study week (Fig. 6.4).

As previously discussed, the use of epidurals is skewed by the fact that in a significant number of units they were not available, or their availability is restricted. In 79 units (28%) no-one had an epidural anaesthetic. If these units are excluded, the average

proportion of women using epidurals was 25%. In some units, the proportion exceeded 50%, although some of this effect might have been due to small number bias (Fig. 6.5).

Pethidine remains a common method of pain relief. Figure 6.6 shows that in most units about half of all women in labour receive pethidine. The distribution of its use is similar to the use of relaxation (Fig. 6.7), although in fact there was no correlation between the use of the two techniques (regression coefficient, $R = 0.06$), unlike the correlation between the use of relaxation and massage ($R = 0.494$; see Fig. 6.8).

> I felt pethidine helped relaxation. Did not relieve the pain. Made me mentally dopey and out of control and less concerned with the pain.

Entonox is the most common method of analgesia, being used in 75% of all labours (Fig. 6.9). It is used significantly less commonly when rates of epidural anaesthesia rise above 50% ($R = 0.25$, $p < 0.001$, Fig. 6.10) but even then it is still used in more than half of all labours.

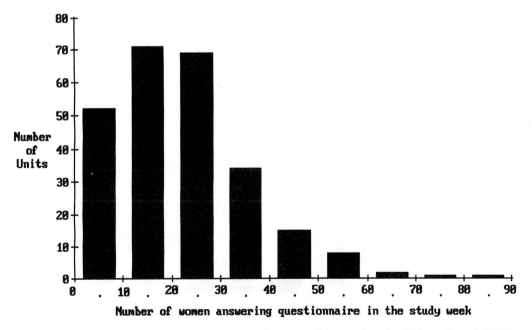

Fig. 6.1 The number of units by the number of women who answered the questionnaires in the study week (NBT 1990).

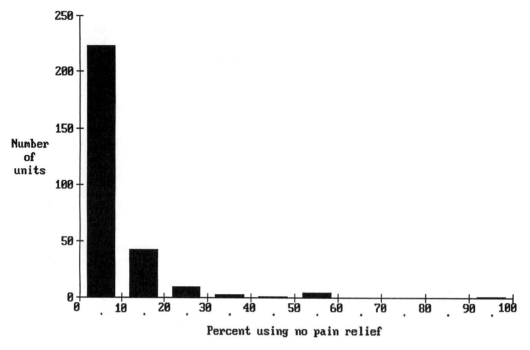

Fig. 6.2 The number of units by the proportions of women reported as using no pain relief (NBT 1990).

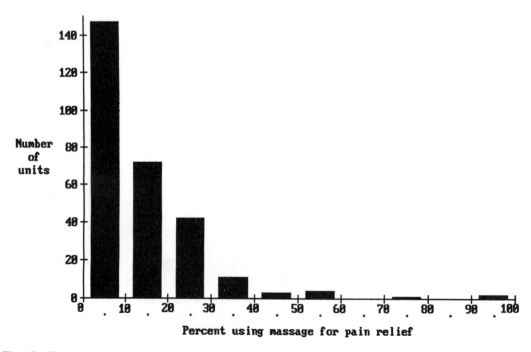

Fig. 6.3 The number of units by the proportions of women reported as using massage for pain relief (NBT 1990).

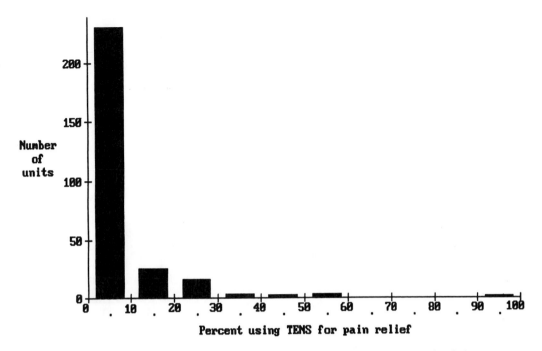

Fig. 6.4 The number of units by the proportions of women reported as using transcutaneous electrical nerve stimulation (TENS) for pain relief (NBT 1990).

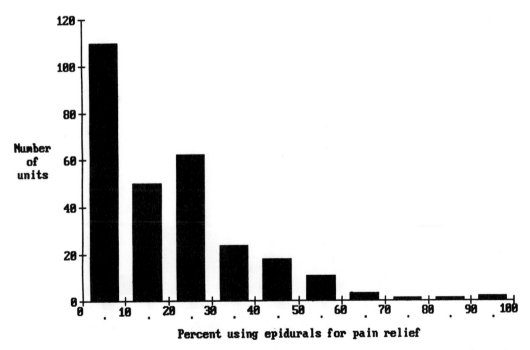

Fig. 6.5 The number of units by the proportions of women reported as using epidural anaesthesia for pain relief (NBT 1990).

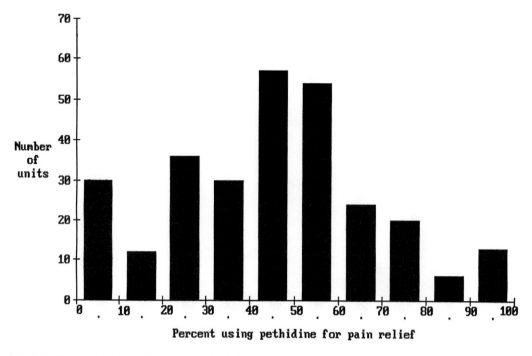

Fig. 6.6   The number of units by the proportions of women reported as using pethidine for pain relief (NBT 1990).

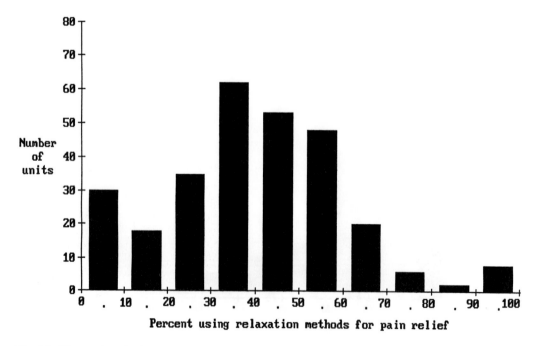

Fig. 6.7   The number of units by the proportions of women reported as using relaxation methods for pain relief (NBT 1990).

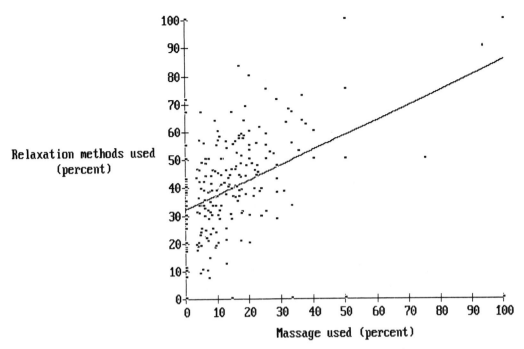

Fig. 6.8 The correlation between the percentages of those using relaxation and those using massage – see text (NBT 1990).

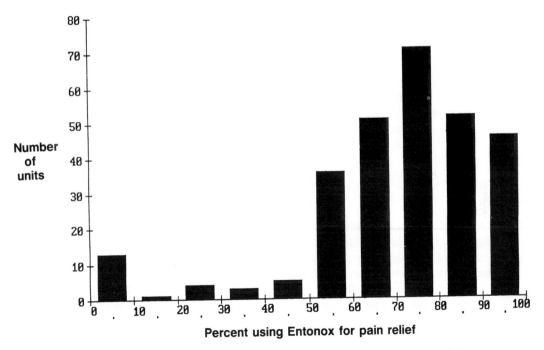

Fig. 6.9 The number of units by the proportions of women reported as using Entonox for pain relief (NBT 1990).

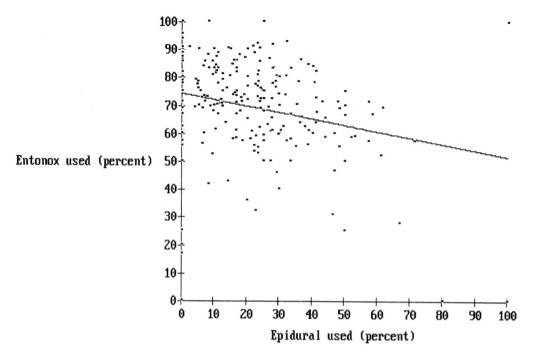

Fig. 6.10   The correlation between the percentage of those using Entonox and those using epidural analgesia (NBT 1990).

Although gas had little effect, it was excellent for calming as my wife had total control of it. It also helped when she was delivering as she could get a good rhythm with her breathing as the mask 'whistled'. (partner's comment)

The use of epidural anaesthesia has a similar but rather more marked effect on the use of pethidine, which falls from almost 50% of all labours to under 30% as the epidural rate rises ($R = 0.39$, $p < 0.0001$; Fig. 6.11).

FACTORS INFLUENCING THE USE OF ANALGESIA

In order to study the factors influencing the overall choice of analgesia in depth, rather than the factors influencing the choice of a particular method such as epidural anaesthesia, it was necessary to construct a theoretical structure which would enable the use of correlation and multivariate analysis. For this purpose, it was assumed that the methods of pain relief lay in a spectrum from none on the one extreme to epidural anaesthesia, the maximum analgesic, on the other. The non-technological methods (no pain relief, relaxation and massage) were grouped together and given a score of 0. TENS was given a score of 1, Entonox 2, pethidine 3 and epidural 4. A method with a higher score was considered to take precedence over a method with a lower score. Thus if a woman used TENS and an epidural, it was assumed that she had moved on from TENS to the epidural, rather than the other way around. Similarly, the use of TENS was considered to take precedence over the use of relaxation. For example, if a woman planned to use TENS and relaxation, her score was 1 for planned analgesia. If she used pethidine and an epidural, her score was 4 for analgesia used. The use of this ranking system was arbitrary but was based on the common conceptions of efficacy widely expressed by women who have used the various methods.

The value of this approach is that it reduced the categories for analgesia in the three-part analysis of what was planned in labour, what was actually used, and what was planned for the next labour to only five. This made analysis much more practical than if the ungrouped methods had been used. If the original seven methods were considered individually, with more than one possible in each labour,

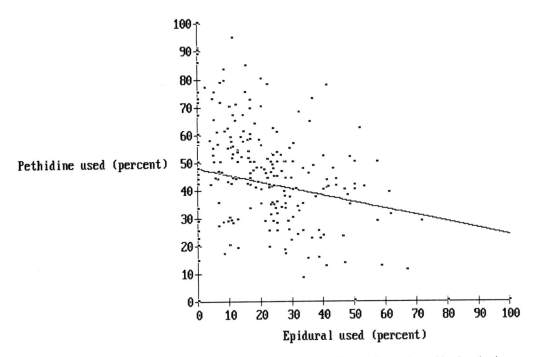

Fig. 6.11   The correlation between the percentage of those using pethidine and those using epidural analgesia (NBT 1990).

there would have been 53 categories, resulting in very small numbers in some of the categories.

Using individual correlation, Table 6.2 shows the most important influences on the method actually used.

However, multivariate analysis showed that the effects of parity and mode of onset of labour operated predominantly through their effect on the duration of labour. Thus, the multiple correlation coefficient of 0.53 was mainly due to the effect of the method planned ($t = 21.9$) and the duration of the first stage of labour ($t = 12.6$), followed by the mode of onset of labour ($t = 8.9$) and parity ($t = 4.9$).

The other factors making a minor contribution to the method of analgesia planned are shown in Table 6.3.

The effects of the duration of labour are shown in Figures 6.12 and 6.13, for the 3978 cases where this variable was recorded.

In nulliparae ($n = 1644$; Fig. 6.14), there is a slow fall, albeit from a very low level, of women using no pain relief or TENS as labour becomes longer. The use of Entonox remains steady at about

Table 6.2   Individual correlation of the most important influences on the method used (NBT Survey 1990)

	R^a
Method planned	0.339
Parity	0.274
Duration of the first stage of labour	0.273
Mode of onset of labour (spontaneous or induced)	0.124

[a]Regression coefficient.

Table 6.3   Factors affecting analgesia used (NBT Survey 1990)

Factor	t^a	p^b
Method planned	21.9	0.0001
Duration of first stage of labour	12.6	0.0001
Mode of onset of labour	8.9	0.0001
Parity	4.9	0.0001
Maximum level of pain experienced	4.8	0.0001
Experience in a previous labour	4.4	0.0001
Advised by a doctor	3.8	0.0001
Antenatal class – other	3.5	0.0005
Antenatal class – hospital	3.2	0.0014
Maternal age	2.6	0.01
Antenatal class – NCT	2.2	0.0263

[a]Student's t-test value.
[b]Probability value.

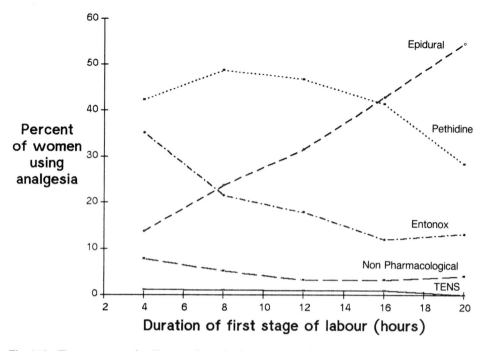

Fig. 6.12   The percentage of nulliparae using a dominant method of analgesia by the duration of labour –
see text (NBT 1990).

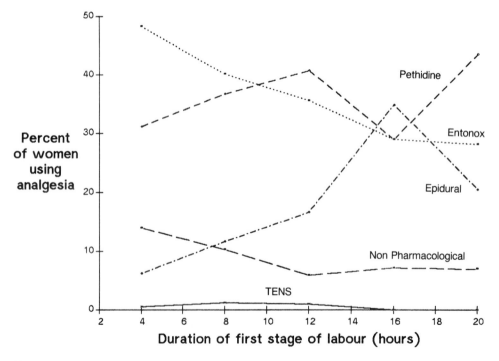

Fig. 6.13   The percentage of multiparae using a dominant method of analgesia by the duration of labour –
see text (NBT 1990).

75%. The use of relaxation and pethidine, on the other hand, shows a small but steady rise. The most marked effect is seen with epidural anaesthesia, which increases from 13.7% in labours lasting up to 4 hours in length, to 54.5% in labours lasting more than 16 hours.

In multiparae (Fig. 6.13), the findings are similar except that there is a lower use of epidural anaesthesia and a higher use of TENS and no pain relief. The use of pethidine is about 10% lower overall, but the use of Entonox remains high and constant at about 75%.

Figure 6.14 shows that when the method of analgesia is plotted by dominant method, the rise in the use of epidural anaesthesia in nulliparae is initially in addition to Entonox, but that after 12 hours it takes over in labours previously managed with pethidine. Figure 6.15 shows a similar effect in multiparae.

Figure 6.16 shows that when labours lasted 4 hours or less, there was no significant difference in the use of pethidine between women using epidural

anaesthesia and those not using epidural anaesthesia. However, in labours lasting 4–12 hours, women not using epidurals were significantly more likely to use pethidine. The use of pethidine in these women increased up to 12 hours, but then plateaued. Interestingly, the percentage of women using pethidine in addition to epidural anaesthesia increased rapidly after 12 hours and actually exceeded that in the non-epidural group after 16 hours. Perhaps this reflects the need for pharmacological support in long labours despite adequate analgesia; alternatively it might represent women giving up the use of pethidine alone and increasingly resorting to the superior effect of epidural anaesthesia.

Table 6.4 shows a direct relation between duration of labour and use of epidural anaesthesia. Overall, nulliparae were about twice as likely to use epidural anaesthesia compared with multiparae.

Induction of labour increased with the proportion of women who chose epidural anaesthesia. Of the 1469 nulliparae who had a spontaneous onset of

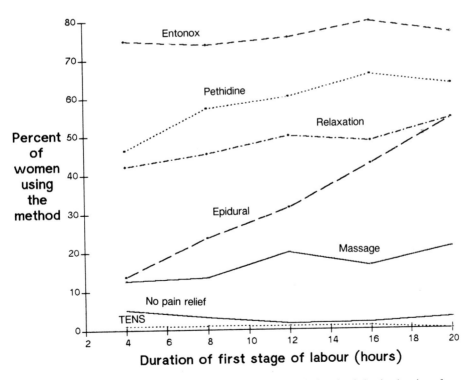

Fig. 6.14 The percentage of nulliparae using non-exclusive method of analgesia by the duration of labour – see text (NBT 1990).

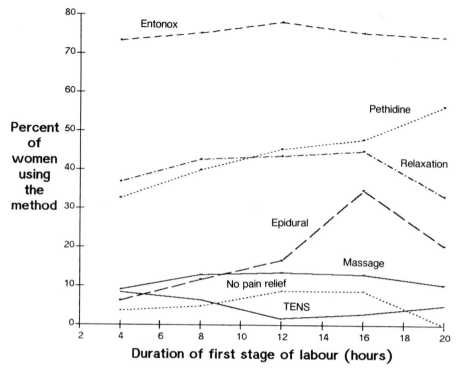

Fig. 6.15 The percentage of multiparae using a non-exclusive method of analgesia by the duration of labour – see text (NBT 1990).

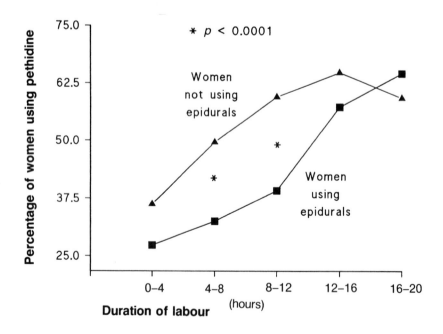

Fig. 6.16 The percentage of women using pethidine who also did or did not use an epidural analgesia by the duration of labour – see text (NBT 1990).

Table 6.4 Percentage of women using epidural anaesthesia during labour (NBT Survey 1990)

Duration of Labour (h)	Nulliparae			Multiparae		
	Total n	No. using epidurals	(%)	Total n	No. using epidurals	(%)
<4	270	37	(13.7)	1007	62	(6.2)
4–7.9	619	147	(23.7)	930	108	(11.6)
8–11.9	438	138	(31.5)	289	48	(16.6)
12–15.9	218	93	(42.7)	69	24	(34.8)
⩾16	99	54	(54.5)	39	8	(20.5)

Table 6.5 How does the method planned affect the method used? (NBT Survey 1990)

636 women (14%) planned to use non-technical (non-pharmacological) methods of pain relief (none, massage, relaxation). Of these:

    203 (32%) succeeded
      4 (0.6%) used TENS
    177 (28%) used Entonox
    184 (29%) used pethidine
     68 (11%) used an epidural

87 (1.97%) women planned to use no more than TENS. Of these:

      4 (5%)   used non-pharmacological methods
     15 (17%) used TENS
     24 (28%) used Entonox
     26 (30%) used pethidine
     18 (21%) used an epidural

1531 (33%) women planned to use no more than Entonox. Of these:

     73 (5%)   used non-pharmacological methods
     15 (17%) used TENS
    821 (54%) used Entonox
    436 (29%) used pethidine
    184 (12%) used an epidural

1588 (34%) women planned to use no more than pethidine. Of these:

     76 (5%)   used non-pharmacological methods
    329 (21%) used Entonox
    958 (60%) used pethidine
    225 (14%) used epidural

812 (17%) women planned to use an epidural. Of these:

     32 (4%)   used non-pharmacological methods
      2 (0.2%) used TENS
    179 (22%) used Entonox
    183 (23%) used pethidine
    416 (51%) used an epidural

spontaneous labour choosing epidurals (8.8%) compared with 112 of the 560 women induced (20%).

Table 6.5 shows that a substantial number of women achieve their ambition in terms of the pain relief they actually use. The proportion was 32% in the case of women wanting to use non-pharmacological methods, 17% in the case of TENS, 54% in the case of Entonox, 60% in the case of pethidine, and 51% in the case of epidurals. Thus the poorest success rates, as might be expected, were with TENS and the non-pharmacological methods, although it is perhaps surprising that fewer succeeded with TENS than without any analgesia at all.

The success of women's intended method can be expressed graphically by computing a variable (called *change*) which is the actual method used minus the intended method, thus:

No pain relief planned (0),
Epidural used (4),
CHANGE = 4.

Pethidine planned (3),
Entonox used (2),
CHANGE = − 1.

Figure 6.17 shows the overall distribution of change. 2341 (51.8%) of women achieved their intended type of analgesia. Figure 6.18 shows the distribution for nulliparae and Figure 6.19 for multiparae. It is evident that more nulliparae move up the analgesia ranking order by one point (419 of 1923, 21.8%) than multiparae (250 of 2593, 9.6%). In fact, multiparae as a group tend slightly to move down. The difference between the two parity groups is highly significant (chi-squared = 221, $p < 0.0001$). This suggests that nulliparae are probably rather over-optimistic in their approach to labour, whereas for multiparae the more rapid labour and easier delivery comes as a welcome surprise.

labour, 385 (26.2%) had an epidural, compared with 173 of 442 (39.1%) following induction of labour. In multiparae, the figures showed an even greater ratio, with only 176 of 2007 women with

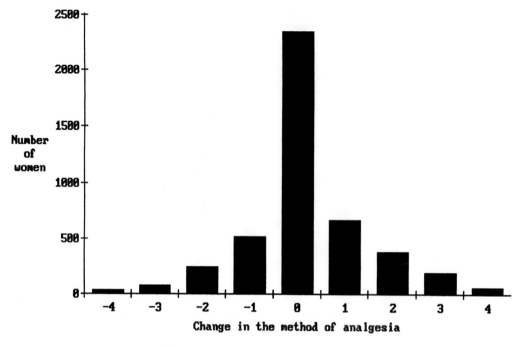

Fig. 6.17   The number of women reporting changes in the method of analgesia – see text (NBT 1990).

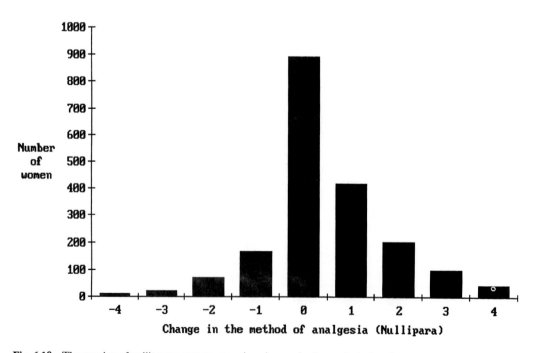

Fig. 6.18   The number of nulliparous women reporting changes in the method of analgesia – see text (NBT 1990).

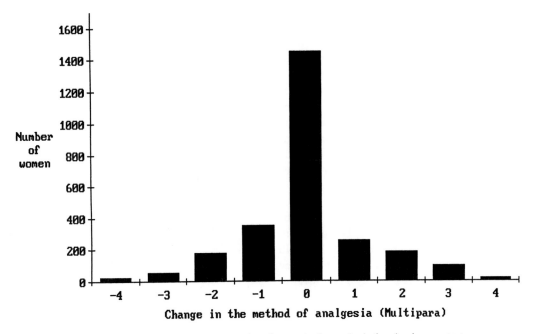

Fig. 6.19 The number of multiparous women reporting changes in the method of analgesia – see text (NBT 1990).

FACTORS AFFECTING THE CHOICE OF PLANNED METHOD

Women obtained their information about pain relief from a wide variety of sources. The source of information had almost no effect on the method chosen. Three sources were just statistically significant in influencing the planned method, although the association was so weak as to be of no practical significance. These were a friend ($n = 1591$, 36% $R = 0.08$), a doctor ($n = 506$, 11%, $R = 0.07$), and previous experience ($n = 1963$, 45%, $R = 0.02$). Other sources of information, in order of frequency mentioned, were books (2468, 55%), antenatal classes (2364, 52%), magazines (1188, 26%) family (797, 18%), television (227, 5%) and newspapers (76, 1.7%).

The type of antenatal classes (Table 6.6) had some effect on the method planned, although again it was very slight.

> I think the parentcraft classes are important and help you to learn and understand about your labour. The breathing and relaxation taught there is thoroughly beneficial. If taught beforehand, they do work.

Table 6.6 Types of antenatal instruction classes attended (NBT Survey 1990)

Type of class	n^a	(%)	R^b	P^c
Health centre	1525	(34)	0.039	0.011
Hospital	1078	(23.9)	0.038	0.013
National Childbirth Trust	194	(4.3)	0.046	0.001
Other classes	44	(1)	0.048	0.001

[a]Total number of women attending.
[b]Regression coefficient.
[c]Probability value.

Frequency of attendance at antenatal classes and correlation with the method of analgesia planned

There were some demographic differences between the women attending the various forms of classes. For example, women attending the National Childbirth Trust (NCT) classes were significantly more likely to be married (90.3%) than those attending the other classes (health centre 77.8%, hospital 78.4%, other 72.7%). The women attending the NCT and other classes were more likely to be multiparous (46.5%) than the health centre (41.4%) or the hospital (38%). There were, however, no differences in the experience of pain in labour, nor their feeling of freedom to choose their method of pain relief, between the four groups.

There were, perhaps as a result of these demographic differences, significant differences in the analgesia choices and use of women who attended the NCT classes, compared to the others (Table 6.7). For example, 10.3% of women attending NCT planned to use TENS as opposed to 6.7% of the others, and 48% planned to use Entonox as opposed to 33%. On the other hand, only 15% planned to use pethidine compared with 35% of the others. Similar proportions planned to use an epidural (15.7% and 17%, respectively) (overall chi-squared 108, $p < 0.0001$).

These preferences were borne out in practice (Table 6.8), with proportions of analgesia used by women attending the NCT being non-pharmacological 13% (vs. 8.2% for the rest), TENS 5.4% (vs. 0.6%), Entonox 38% (vs. 33%), pethidine 21% (vs. 40%) and epidurals 23% (vs. 19%) (overall chi-squared 73, $p < 0.0001$). Similar proportions were intended in the next pregnancy (Table 6.9), being non-pharmacological 11% (vs. 6%), TENS 5% (vs. 1%), Entonox 39% (vs. 28%), pethidine 14.6% (vs. 36%) and epidurals 31% (vs. 29.6%) (overall chi-squared 59, $p < 0.0001$).

The small number of women attending other classes were also atypical. 28% planned to use non-pharmacological (vs. 13.5% for the rest) and 11.6% TENS (vs. 1.7%) (chi-squared 32, $p < 0.0001$), and this pattern persisted during labour and into the preferences for the next pregnancy.

> In the classes, I do not think the amount of pain that my wife would suffer was emphasised enough. The impression was given that the pain would be bad but bearable if pethidine was used. This turned out not to be the case.

THE RELATIONSHIP BETWEEN MODE OF DELIVERY AND ANALGESIA IN LABOUR

The relationship between the method of analgesia used and the mode of delivery is always a difficult

Table 6.7 Women (%) planning to use the various methods of pain relief by dominant method (NBT Survey 1990)

Classes	Non-pharm.	TENS	Entonox	Pethidine	Epidural
Health Centre	10.5	2.2	35.6	34.8	16.9
Hospital	10.2	2.6	35.2	33.4	18.6
NCT	11.4	10.3	47.6	15.1	15.7
Other class	27.9	11.6	25.6	20.9	14.0

Table 6.8 Women (%) using the various methods of pain relief by dominant method (NBT Survey 1990)

Classes	Non-pharm.	TENS	Entonox	Pethidine	Epidural
Health Centre	6.6	0.8	27.7	42.7	22.2
Hospital	5.6	1.2	28.9	37.6	26.6
NCT	13.0	5.4	37.8	21.1	22.7
Other class	27.9	4.7	30.2	14.0	23.3

Table 6.9 Women (%) planning to use the various methods of pain relief in the next labour by dominant method (NBT Survey 1990)

Classes	Non-pharm.	TENS	Entonox	Pethidine	Epidural
Health Centre	5.2	1.4	26.1	36.1	31.3
Hospital	5.2	1.3	27.0	29.5	37.0
NCT	10.8	4.9	38.9	14.6	30.8
Other class	21.4	2.4	33.3	16.7	26.2

one to disentangle. The method of analgesia may affect the mode of delivery; for example, epidural anaesthesia is widely cited as increasing the incidence of forceps delivery. A long or particularly painful labour is likely to be associated with both an increased use of analgesia and with instrumental delivery. Thus there is an association between the two which is not necessarily causal.

None the less, observations can be made about the relationship which may have some value, at least as a starting point to develop hypotheses which may be susceptible to proper prospective testing.

When considering mode of delivery, it is first important to be aware that parity has a major influence. Thus in the subset analysis, from which elective Caesareans, multiple pregnancies and breech presentations have been excluded, only 77% of nulliparae delivered spontaneously, compared with 95% of multiparae. The emergency Caesarean section rate was 5.8% in nulliparae compared with only 2% of multiparae.

Nulliparae

The method of analgesia planned had no significant correlation with mode of delivery. When epidurals were planned there was a slight fall in the incidence of spontaneous delivery from an average of 78% to 67%, and and a slight increase in the incidence of non-rotational forceps from 10% to 14.6%, rotational forceps from 2% to 4.6% and Caesarean section from 5% to 7.4%, but these changes were not significant with the numbers in this subset of the study. Such slight changes are entirely consistent with the possibility that in higher risk labours the mother or her medical attendants anticipated problems and chose a more potent method of analgesia accordingly.

There was, however, a highly significant association between the method actually used and the mode of delivery (chi-squared = 255, p <0.0001). All 17 women using TENS delivered spontaneously, compared with 85.5–88% of women using non-pharmacological methods, Entonox or pethidine, and only 55% of women using epidurals. This was probably due to the effect of prolonged labour on both the method of analgesia (see before) and the mode of delivery – the spontaneous delivery rate fell from 83% to 59.6% as labour went from under 4 hours to over 16, the forceps rate increased from 10% to 20% (non-rotational) and 1.5% to 4% (rotational), the ventouse rate from 3% to 5.1%, and the Caesarean section rate from 2.2% to 11.1%.

The mode of delivery was reflected in the choice of analgesia for the next labour. The planned use of epidural rose from 29% after a spontaneous occipito-anterior delivery, to 45% after a spontaneous occipito-posterior delivery, 53% after a non-rotational forceps, 72.5% after a rotational forceps, and 69.4% after an emergency Caesarean (Fig. 6.20).

Multiparae

The effects described above for nulliparae also occurred with multiparae, but are not so clearly demonstrable due to the small numbers having instrumental and operative deliveries.

OTHER FACTORS INFLUENCING CHOICE AND USE OF ANALGESIA

Ethnic origin

Most factors other than duration of labour, parity and method of onset have a very small effect. Ethnic origin had some effect but the numbers of ethnic minority women in the study were too small to draw clear conclusions. 94% (4272) of the subset population were white, 1.1% (50) Indian, 0.8% (37) Afro-Caribbean black, 0.6% (27) African black, 0.7% (33) Pakistani, 0.2% (11) Chinese and 0.2%

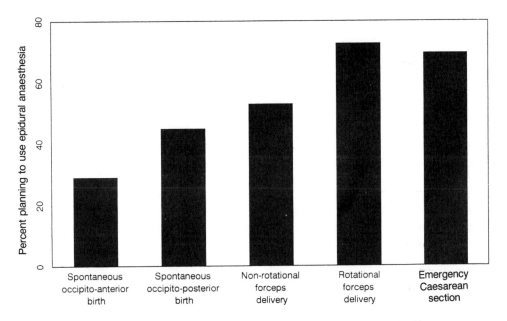

Fig. 6.20 The planned use of analgesia in the next pregnancy by the mode of delivery in this pregnancy (NBT 1990).

(7) Bangladeshi while 63 were of other race. Thus it is only possible to make tentative comments about the first five of these groups.

Pakistani women were most likely to plan non-pharmacological methods (39%), followed by Africans (37%), Indians (30%), Afro-Caribbeans (16%) and whites (13%). Only two non-white women chose TENS (one Afro-Caribbean and one Chinese). Indian and Pakistani women were less likely to plan Entonox (24% and 14%, respectively) than white, African or Afro-Caribbean (34%, 35% and 37%, respectively). Indian and African women were also less likely to plan pethidine (20% and 15%, respectively) than white, Afro-Caribbean and Pakistani women (35%, 30% and 30% respectively). The percentages planning epidurals ranged from 11% (black) through 16% (Afro-Caribbean), 17% (white), 18% (Pakistani) to 26% (Indian).

In terms of analgesia used, this largely reflected parity. The highly parous Indians and Pakistanis managed to use non-pharmacological methods in 18% and 27% of labours respectively, compared with 7% of Africans, 8% of whites and none of the Afro-Caribbeans. The use of Entonox and pethidine was fairly similar in all groups, as was the use of epidurals (the lowest figure being 15% in the Pakistanis and the highest 24% in the Afro-Caribbeans).

Freedom of choice

The woman's feeling of freedom of choice presented an intriguing finding. Overall, 2961 (66.5%) felt very free in their choice, 1147 (25.8%) fairly free, 238 (5.3%) not very free and only 105 (2.5%) not at all free. The reasons they did not feel free were not recorded and might, for example, be related more to anticipated medical complications than social restraint. The planning of epidurals increased from 15.5% if the woman felt very free to 34% if she was not at all free (chi-squared = 74.5, $p < 0.0001$) but interestingly in actual use the epidural rate decreased from 20.8% when the woman felt very free to 12.4% when she did not feel at all free (chi-squared = 86.7, $p < 0.0001$). Perhaps this reflects a desire to have an epidural which is frustrated by a lack of availability.

> I feel it is almost impossible to make the right personal decision about pain relief before having experienced a complete labour. Before then, you just do not know what to expect. This was my second labour and I knew what choices I wanted to make. Knowledge is the key.

Marital status

Marital status (75.8% were married) had no effect at all on planned analgesia, but married women were slightly more likely to use non-pharmacological methods (9.1% vs. 6.5%).

Partner present

163 women said they were alone in labour, but this affected neither the method of analgesia planned nor that used. Women having their husband present (3936, 87%) were less likely to use non-pharmacological methods (7.8% vs. 12.6%) and more likely to use epidurals (19.4% vs. 15.7%). Similar increases in epidural usage were seen in women having other family members present (22.6% vs 18.5%), and when the midwife was present throughout labour, as she was in 1730 (38%) cases (19.2% vs. 18.7%).

Suggestions as to the pain relief which might be used mostly came from the women themselves (46%) and the midwife (47%). In 4.2% it was the partner's suggestion, in 1.3% that of the obstetrician, and in only 0.4% that of the anaesthetist.

HOW DID CHOICE OF ANALGESIA AFFECT PERCEPTIONS OF PAIN IN LABOUR?

One of the questions asked women to state whether in labour there were times when she was 'pain free', 'in mild pain', 'in severe pain' or 'in unbearable pain'. The answers to these questions have been recoded so that the maximum pain experienced in labour is the final variable. For example, a woman never experiencing pain in labour at any time was considered pain free, whereas a woman saying she was at any time in severe pain was coded as having severe pain, even if there were times she was pain free.

Only 2.1% of women said they were pain free throughout labour. 4.4% said they experienced mild pain, 37.5% severe pain and 56% unbearable pain. These findings have important implications for counselling in antenatal classes. 93.5% of women say they have severe or unbearable pain in labour despite the widespread use of analgesia; labour is clearly an extremely painful experience for the overwhelming majority of women and it is unrealistic to obfuscate this painful fact.

If anything, labour was slightly less painful when it was induced (3.2% saying they had no pain vs. 1.8% in spontaneous labour, and 91.7% severe or unbearable pain vs. 94% in spontaneous labour), but the difference was only marginally significant (chi-squared = 10, p = 0.016).

The likelihood of unbearable pain increased significantly with prolonged labour, from 49.6% in labours less than 4 hours to 65% in labours longer than 16 hours (chi-squared = 44.6, $p < 0.0001$).

The method of analgesia used also had a slight effect on the level of pain. Pain was severe or unbearable in 92.2% of women using non-pharmacological methods, 97.2% of women using TENS, 94.3% of women using Entonox, 95.3% of women using pethidine, and 88.9% of those using epidurals. However, women using non-pharmacological methods and TENS were less likely to complain of unbearable pain (33%) than those using Entonox (53%), pethidine (63%) or epidurals (59%) (chi-squared = 186, $p < 0.0001$).

CONCLUSIONS

The methods of pain relief planned and used in labour are affected only slightly by the sources of advice. Rather, the choice is a personal one and is mostly modified by experience in a previous birth, and the mode of onset and duration of labour. Most women have a reasonable chance of succeeding with their planned method of pain relief. The experience of severe pain in labour, however, remains an overwhelmingly common experience despite the use of analgesia.

7. Obstetrical anaesthesia

M. Morgan

In the relief of pain in childbirth, a wide variety of drugs and routes of application are used by obstetricians and obstetric anaesthetists. This chapter is concerned mostly, however, with those methods which need the skills of an anaesthetist – epidural analgesia and general anaesthesia.

Although some obstetricians have been trained to give epidural anaesthetics, in the UK it is customary to use the skills of a specialist anaesthetist to do this as no obstetrician should have to be responsible for dealing with complications that might arise from the epidural and from the mother or fetus coincidentally.

EPIDURAL ANALGESIA

Epidural analgesia in obstetrics, via the caudal route, was thought to have been performed first in the US in 1942, but the German anaesthetist Stoeckel used the method on a few women in the early 1900s; continuous caudal analgesia was first used by the Rumanian, Aburel, in 1931. The method was slow to develop in the UK and did not become popular until the late 1960s but is now available to many women in labour in this country. There were many problems with the caudal access at the bottom of the sacrum and so lumbar epidural analgesia has replaced it and is now used almost exclusively. Here the anaesthetic is introduced into the area around the nerves as they leave the spinal cord between two lumbar vertebrae.

Placement of an epidural catheter requires considerable technical skill and therefore there must be trained staff in adequate numbers to provide the service. Lack of anaesthetists is usually the limiting factor for a 24 h epidural service.

Injecting the correct amount of local anaesthetic into the right part of the epidural space should completely abolish the pains of labour, but can also be accompanied by potentially serious complications. A mother having an epidural anaesthetic requires constant observation and the price of this superior pain relief is a marked increase in the workload of skilled midwives and anaesthetists.

The present study reports the results of the first large-scale consumer investigation of the use of epidural analgesia in labour in the United Kingdom.

Availability of epidural analgesia

As small isolated maternity units continue to close throughout the UK, more births are taking place in the larger consultant units (see Ch. 4). Following this trend, epidural analgesia is now becoming available to many more women for pain relief in labour and not just for strictly medical indications as it used to be.

> In a previous labour my wife had the benefit of an epidural which was very successful – indeed so much so that I cannot understand why this is not more freely available. The contrast between the first labour with an epidural and the second one without was immense.

The proportion of units in each region providing an epidural service and those providing that service over the full 24-hour period can be been in Table 7.1 and Figure 7.1. In those regions where many isolated units still exist – e.g. Scotland, South Western and West Midlands – the availability of epidural analgesia is obviously lower than in such regions as South West Thames where all maternity services are provided in medium and large units.

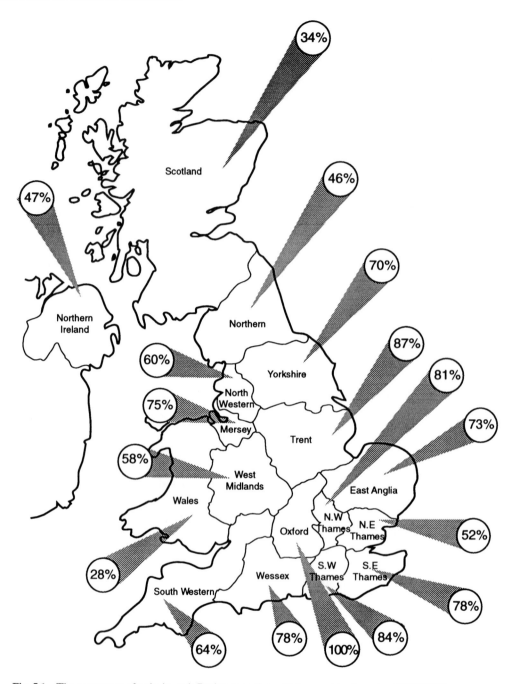

Fig. 7.1 The percentage of units in each Region reporting a 24-hour epidural service (NBT 1990).

Parity

Of the 10 351 women in the study, 2290 (22%) received epidural analgesia. These included 1146 of the 4445 primiparous (26%) but only 844 of the 5906 multiparous women (14%).

This trend is consistent with the many smaller studies with about half as many primiparous as multiparous women having an epidural. Lower levels of pain and shorter labours in the multiparous are influences while the later arrival of the

Table 7.1 Regional availability of epidurals by proportion of units providing epidural analgesia (NBT Survey 1990)

Region	Epidural available (%)	24-hour service available (%)
Northern	84	46
Yorkshire	88	70
Trent	93	87
East Anglia	82	73
North West Thames	87	81
North East Thames	73	52
South East Thames	78	78
South West Thames	100	84
Wessex	78	78
Oxford	100	100
South Western	64	64
West Midlands	58	58
Mersey	87	75
North Western	70	60
Channel Islands	100	100
Northern Ireland	60	47
Scotland	47	34
Wales	40	28
Armed Services	100	100
Independent	100	100

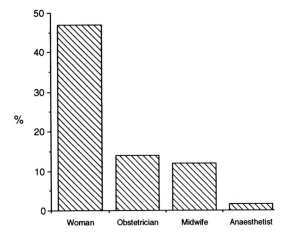

Fig. 7.2 The percentage of women having epidural anaesthesia by who decided on the method (NBT 1990).

decision in a very small number of instances (0.17%); the GP was at a similar level (0.2%).

Uptake of epidural analgesia

According to the women who participated in the study, 1175 (18%) used epidural analgesia as a method of pain relief during their labour and the birth of their baby. These have been identified by region and comparisons made with the number of deliveries where epidural was used in the NBT Survey 1984 where again data were based on the women's reports (see Table 7.3 and Fig. 7.3). The epidural rate has increased in 12 of the 17 regions compared, remained the same in one, and decreased in four. This decrease is a point of concern, for elsewhere we show women's overall satisfaction with the method. It is unlikely that the women of East Anglia or Mersey have changed their minds so much in 6 years.

To assess if this was associated with a cutback in anaesthetists, we checked the data for consultant anaesthetists available in the day reported to the 1984 and 1990 surveys. This is only one measure of the problem as consultants are not the only anaesthetists giving epidurals and many such procedures are done at night rather than in the day only. The number of units has diminished in the 6 year gap but both sets of data are given as percentages. These are coarse figures but when doing national volunteer questionnaire surveys one is sketching with broad figures and not fine data

multiparous in hospital in the labour process may also contribute to this reduced usage.

Decision to use an epidural

The person who made the decision to use epidural analgesia, as reported by the midwives, is shown in Table 7.2. and Figure 7.2. On the majority of occasions this was by the woman alone (47%) or in conjunction with the midwife (17%). The midwife alone recommended the method to 281 women (12%) and the obstetrician alone to 318 women (14%). The partner alone was involved in the

Table 7.2 Decision to start epidural anaesthesia (NBT Survey 1990)

	n	(%)
Woman	1101	(47)
Midwife	281	(12)
Obstetrician	318	(14)
Anaesthetist	37	(1.6)
General Practitioner	5	(0.2)
Partner	4	(0.2)
Other	3	(0.1)
Woman plus midwife	407	(17)
Other combinations of above	191	(8)

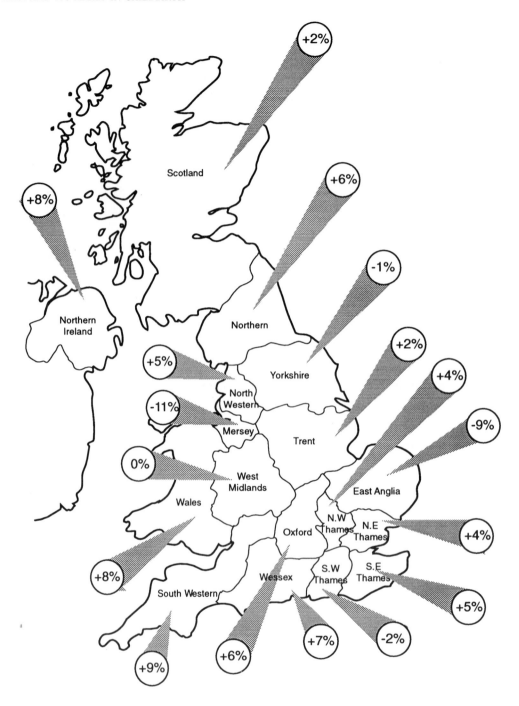

Fig. 7.3   The difference in percentages of women in each Region using epidural anaesthesia between the NBT studies of 1984 and 1990 by Region.

Table 7.3 Women's observations of the use of epidural analgesia (NBT Survey 1984 and 1990)

Region	Deliveries for which an epidural was given (%)		
	1984	1990	Difference
Northern	11	17	+ 6
Yorkshire	23	22	− 1
Trent	20	22	+ 2
East Anglia	27	18	− 9
North West Thames	24	28	+ 4
North East Thames	9	13	+ 4
South East Thames	14	19	+ 5
South West Thames	20	18	− 2
Wessex	11	18	+ 7
Oxford	15	21	+ 6
South Western	15	24	+ 9
West Midlands	18	18	0
Mersey	30	19	− 11
North Western	12	17	+ 5
Channel Islands	NK	13	NK
Northern Ireland	6	14	+ 8
Scotland	18	20	+ 2
Wales	8	16	+ 8
Armed Services	NK	19	NK
Independent	NK	54	NK

NK, not known.

methods. It seems, from comparison of Table 7.3, that in nine Regions there has been an increased proportion of consultant anaesthetists, while in eight there was a reduction, notably South West Thames and Mersey. There was, however, little correlation between the two sets of data as there were increased epidural rates in Thames Regions, North Western and Wales despite lower anaesthetist staffing rates; in East Anglia and Mersey, despite both Regions reporting increased staffing levels of anaesthetists, there were few epidurals available.

Complicated labour

The number of mothers reported to have hypertensive disease, multiple pregnancy or breech presentation and who received an epidural are shown in Table 7.4.

There are possible beneficial effects to a mother and baby of an epidural analgesia if a woman with hypertensive disease is in labour. Further, because of the occasional need for sudden and unexpected interventions in twin and breech deliveries, many obstetricians find a well supervised continuous and

Table 7.4. Women with complicated pregnancies having epidurals (NBT Survey 1990)

Complication	Total no. in study	No. having epidurals	(%)
Hypertensive disease	842	274	(33)
Multiple pregnancy	104	55	(53)
Breech presentation	368	63	(17)

effective epidural anaesthetic a wise precaution. The proportions who had this help is disappointing, particularly for those with hypertensive disease and breech delivery. It may be that with the wider medical management of the former with rapidly acting antihypertensive and anticonvulsive agents the indication for an epidural anaesthetic is now thought by obstetricians to be less strong.

> Although I was against having an epidural through fear of scare stories and injections, I am extremely grateful I took the hospital's advice as I had high blood pressure and then a forceps delivery.

Gestation

The duration of gestation at the time of epidural analgesia is shown in Table 7.5, together with the gestation at delivery of all the women in the study. Again it would seem that there was a disappointingly low usage of epidurals in many of the more preterm cases. The preterm low birth weight infant is highly sensitive to the depressant effects of pethidine and other narcotic agents so that benefits may follow their avoidance. Inside small figure variation, in pregnancies finishing before 37 weeks, over twice as many fetuses were exposed to narcotic agents (5.4%) than to the effects of an epidural

Table 7.5 Duration of gestation of women having an epidural (NBT Survey 1990)

Gestation (weeks)	No. in study n	Epidural n	(%)	GA and narcotic agents n	(%)
<24	3	1	—	0	(0)
24–28	27	3	(11)	13	(48)
29–32	91	21	(23)	59	(65)
33–36	426	115	(27)	225	(53)
37–40	7055	1517	(22)	3856	(55)
41–42	2407	583	(24)	1470	(61)
>42	14	4	—	7	(50)
TOTAL	10 023	2244	(24)	5630	

(2.5%). Allowing for the percentage of women who received all three methods recorded, detailed breakdown shows an increased frequency of women in labour with very small babies receiving pethidine rather than epidural.

Method of delivery

The mode of delivery in those who had an epidural anaesthetic is shown in Table 7.6. The study confirms the higher spontaneous delivery rate among multiparae who had an epidural compared with nulliparae. The combined operative vaginal delivery rate of primiparae and multiparae who had epidurals was 23.4%, compared to 6% among the women who did not have them. Even allowing for the fact that epidural anaesthesia would have been used in some women because of the likelihood of operative delivery, these figures would seem to favour a likely association of vaginal instrumental delivery with an epidural.

The Caesarean section rate in women without an epidural was 8%, compared with an overall survey rate of 11.4%. These values are slightly lower than the national average, but probably within the normal fluctuation rate over a period of one week. In the other groups epidural analgesia would have been used electively for many of the Caesarean sections.

Effectiveness of pain relief

The results of the different forms of pain relief are shown in Table 7.7. Although the effectiveness of analgesia was assessed by midwives, obstetricians, anaesthetists, partners and the women concerned, the results of the latter are presented here, for in many ways it is the perceived pain noted by the

woman that really matters rather than seeking to find some Eldorado of objective measures.

The results confirm that epidural anaesthesia produces analgesia superior to any other technique, with very good (75%) or good (18%) pain relief being reported by 93% of women. 89% reported positively after relaxation and breathing exercises and 84% with Entonox. Only 72% seemed so positive about pethidine and 75% with TENS.

Complications

The complications are reported in Table 7.8; figures for these will be only those of a short term nature in Branch 2 for reporting was soon after delivery; 6-week comments are found in the postal follow-up in Chapter 10. The commonest problem was hypotension, accounting for 61% of the complications reported in the epidural group. Set in context this implies hypotension in 2.3% of the 2290 women who had an epidural.

Among those who had an epidural anaesthetic, dural puncture was reported in 11 women, a rate of just 0.5%, a lower proportion than reported in some earlier studies. Again, the nature of the study did not allow for the full reporting of post-dural puncture headache in Branch 2 but is considered in Branch 3.

CAESAREAN SECTION

Caesarean section was performed on 1151 women, of whom just half had regional anaesthesia (459 epidural and 6 spinal anaesthetics). 284 mothers were already having an epidural through a catheter into the epidural space when the decision was made to deliver by Caesarean section.

> I appreciated the talk with the anaesthetist prior to the Caesarean section. I would not hesitate to recommend the epidural method to anyone who was unsure about the total block effect and feeling pain. I think the recovery period afterwards is a great deal better than with a general anaesthetic.

By using regional anaesthesia, difficulties in tracheal intubation and inhalation of gastric contents were avoided; these are the major contributory factors from general anaesthesia to maternal mortality.

Table 7.6 Method of delivery of those having epidurals (NBT Survey 1990)

Method of delivery	Primiparae		Multiparae	
	n	(%)	n	(%)
Spontaneous vertex	646	(46.2)	439	(52.4)
Breech (all)	30	(2.2)	34	(4.1)
Forceps and vacuum extraction	425	(30.4)	98	(11.7)
Elective Caesarean section	95	(6.8)	180	(21.5)
Emergency Caesarean section	201	(14.4)	83	(9.9)
Other and not known	1	(0)	4	(0.4)
TOTAL	1398	100	838	100

Table 7.7 Effectiveness of pain relief assessed by women (NBT Survey 1990)

Assessment	Relaxation		Massage		Tens		Entonox		Pethidine		Epidural	
	n	(%)	n	%	n	%	n	%	n	%	n	%
Very good	690	(35)	426	(38)	80	(25)	1306	(37)	547	(27)	838	(75)
Good	1071	(54)	607	(54)	162	(50)	1650	(47)	921	(45)	205	(18)
Poor	178	(9)	67	(6)	52	(16)	367	(11)	373	(18)	44	(4)
No use	53	(3)	31	(3)	29	(9)	173	(5)	218	(11)	26	(2)

Table 7.8 Incidence of complications after epidural anaesthesia (NBT Survey 1990)

Complication	Total no. reported	No. with epidural
Hypotension	95	54
Vomiting	15	6
Dural tap	11	11
Dyspnoea	1	0
Other	4	3

> Having an anaesthetic for my first Caesarean, I found the epidural a definite improvement as I was able to be awake for the birth of my second child. It was a wonderful experience.

Ethnic origin

The ethnic origin of the mother is shown in Table 7.9. The proportion receiving epidural anaesthesia mirrors the proportion from that particular ethnic class in the study as a whole. The vast majority of women (93%) who had epidurals were white but the proportional results do not suggest that epidural analgesia is being used less frequently by the minority ethnic groups.

Social class

The proportion of women from social classes I, II and IIIN receiving epidural anaesthesia (50%) was slightly greater as a percentage of the total number in those groups in the study, compared with those

Table 7.9 Percentages of women by ethnic origin who received an epidural compared to total in study (NBT Survey 1990)

Ethnic origin	Total study (%)	With epidural (%)
White	92.0	93.0
Black	2.1	2.3
Asian	4.7	4.2
Other	1.3	1.0

in classes IIIM, IV and V (18%). However, the differences between the latter and the total respective class numbers is too small to draw any significant inferences.

Repeat epidurals

Table 7.10 and Figure 7.4 show the opinions of mothers about epidural anaesthesia in a future confinement.

Almost half of those who did not have an epidural would request one in a subsequent confinement, while 35% would not. Of the mothers who had an epidural, 88% would want one in a future labour, and only 6% would not. Questionnaires were also returned by 78 mothers in Branch 3 who had delivered in units with no epidural service. 63 (81%) of these were satisfied or very satisfied with the pain relief they had received, while nine were dissatisfied or very dissatisfied. 74 (95%) of these women would choose the same unit for their next confinement (see Ch. 10).

In addition to the above, 20 women had a forceps delivery under general anaesthesia. This number is small and the exact circumstances are unknown, but even this procedure rarely needs such an anaesthetic nowadays unless, as happens occasionally, the epidural fails as an adequate method of pain relief.

GENERAL ANAESTHESIA

General anaesthesia was used in 49% of women who had a Caesarean section and for a very small

Table 7.10 Opinions of women about epidural analgesia in a future confinement (NBT Survey 1990)

Opinion	No epidural this labour		Epidural this labour	
	n	(%)	n	(%)
Want epidural next labour	1764	(49)	951	(88)
Do not want epidural next labour	1266	(35)	59	(6)
Don't know	547	(16)	62	(6)
TOTAL	3577		1072	

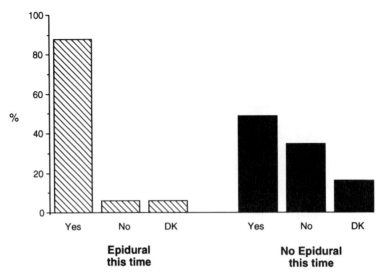

Figure 7.4 The percentage of women who wished to use an epidural anaesthetic in a future confinement by their use of epidural anaethesia on this occasion (DK = Do not know) (NBT 1990).

number of forceps deliveries. The gradual reduction in the use of general anaesthesia nationally reflects the belief that regional anaesthesia is safer for mother and baby; unfortunately it is not possible to perform a controlled trial to confirm this. However, there will always be a need for general anaesthesia, whose great advantages are speed, reliability and controllability. It will be indicated for those mothers who refuse regional anaesthesia, and those with derangements of blood clotting, e.g. in the presence of eclampsia or fulminating pre-eclampsia. There are also the very small number of women for whom very rapid delivery is required for fetal reasons, e.g. in the event of a prolapsed cord. The major problems of general anaesthesia are related to failed tracheal intubation and aspiration of gastric contents at induction of anaesthesia. The former is due to the anatomical configuration of the patient, about which nothing can be done; if, however, an anaesthetist knows of this preoperatively, he is forewarned and everything can be at hand immediately to deal with the situation, including ensuring that senior help is present. Problems mainly occur with unexpected difficult intubation. It is essential that there be a *failed intubation protocol* known to everyone – midwives, anaesthetists and obstetricians. This must be practised, for the first time the failed intubation procedure is used should not be the first time the anaesthetist has to use it.

One section of Branch 2B (Questions 20–22; see Appendix) applied to women who had had a Caesarean section. They were asked to state the type of anaesthetic given, the person who discussed this method with them and whether they were aware of any feelings or sensations during the operation if general anaesthesia was the method used.

Table 7.11 shows that in almost 55% of cases a discussion on the choice of anaesthetic method took place between the woman and a member of the medical staff; in over 30% it was the midwife and 36% the obstetrician, but over 12% of women stated that no discussion had occurred at all. Of the 440 women who reported a general anaesthetic for the Caesarean section, 22 stated that they had been aware of pain, 11 aware of touch and 15 aware of people during the anaesthetic. There is no corrobo-

Table 7.11 Professional who discussed the anaesthetic method as reported by the women (NBT Survey 1990)

Professional	n	(%)
Obstetrician	373	(36.5)
Anaesthetist	141	(13.8)
GP	47	(4.6)
Midwife	314	(30.7)
No-one	125	(12.2)
Other	22	(2.2)
TOTAL	1022	

oration of these symptoms from the anaesthetist within the context of the survey.

CONCLUSIONS

This study has revealed that epidural analgesia is being used for a large number of deliveries in the UK; if this survey week's data can be extrapolated, about 116 000 women will receive an epidural in labour every year. The quality of analgesia provided is superior to that of all other methods and its acceptance by mothers is evidenced by the propor-

tion of women (88%) who would choose the method again for a future confinement, as well as by the percentage (49%) who did not have an epidural for this labour but would choose one in future. The increasing trend to perform Caesarean section under regional anaesthesia is confirmed (51%) and should encouraged. The number of reported complications is low. Epidural analgesia should continue to be available for labour in all women who require and request it but this will depend on the availability of trained anaesthetists in sufficient numbers at each place of confinement.

8. Coping with pain

A. Wraight

Analysis of the responses obtained allowed us to build a picture of the effectiveness of pain relief and to assess a group of other factors that also affected relaxation. Further examination of special groups included those who had home deliveries or gave birth to stillborn babies. A separate analysis of perineal pain was made, for this is sometimes overlooked in analgesia services yet is probably the more common site of pain and problems in the puerperium.

COMPARISON OF EFFECTIVENESS OF PAIN RELIEF METHODS

In her book *A Savage enquiry*, Wendy Savage asks: 'Is there a gulf between what women are seeking in order to control pain and what the professionals want to provide?'

An important part of the analysis of this study was to compare the woman's assessment of her pain relief methods with those who were supporting her in labour – her partner and those who were providing her care, the midwives and doctors. Everyone – the woman, her partner, the midwife, the obstetrician and the anaesthetist – was asked to give their opinion of each method used by ranking it from 'Very good' to 'No use' (see Appendix, Branch 1).

Non-pharmacological methods

In Table 8.1, the main non-pharmacological methods of pain relief used are shown. The totals all relate to 'Very good' and 'Good' assessments which have been combined for this chapter. In the individual assessments from the midwife, woman and partner, the data relate to all the evaluations made but may not be referring to the same labours. The combined column, however, only shows the cases where all three people have agreed that that method was 'Very good' or 'Good' for that particular woman. It can be seen that, in the majority of cases, the women, their partners and the midwives are in agreement.

The discrepancy seen in the number of cases where relaxation exercises and massage were used (363 vs. 1761) according to the midwife and those identified by the women was surprising. Perhaps some midwives felt that these alternative methods were not worthy of mention if the woman was also using a pharmacological form of pain relief. Perhaps some do not consider these as actual pain-relieving techniques, as one partner commented:

> I think there is a difference between pain relief and coping with pain. Relaxation and breathing is a good way of coping with pain without necessarily relieving it.

Table 8.1 Non-pharmacological methods of pain relief assessed as 'Very good' or 'Good' (NBT Survey 1990)

Method	Midwife		Woman		Partner		Midwives, women and partners	
	n	(%)	n	(%)	n	(%)	n	(%)
Relaxation	363	(92)	1761	(88)	844	(87)	51	(89)
Massage	422	(87)	1033	(91)	755	(88)	70	(88)
TENS	309	(74)	242	(75)	203	(75)	112	(79)

Transcutaneous electrical nerve stimulation (TENS) was less useful. This might have been due to practical or technical problems, or lack of adequate preparation. There were detailed accounts of leads becoming disconnected, batteries running out, and machines not being available. Some women had to discontinue its use when internal fetal monitoring was commenced for the equipment interfered with the pick-up of the electronic signal reflected from the fetus. Some partners felt that TENS interfered with back massage. One woman remarked:

> I wanted to try TENS this time but was told that I should have started it immediately on admission. I had not been told this before.

Many women, however, found it very beneficial, especially in the early stages of labour:

> Using the TENS machine for the first time was very good. I was able to cope until late stage without gas and so felt as though I was more in control.

Pharmacological methods

Table 8.2 takes the same form as Table 8.1, but this time giving the main pharmacological methods used. Figure 8.1 illustrates data from the combined column (midwives, women and partners) from Tables 8.1 and 8.2.

Inhalational analgesia was the most widely used method and most women found it helpful – not so much as a pain relieving method but as a distraction and an activity which assisted in relaxation and breathing exercises. Some found it disorientating and with no effect on the pain:

Table 8.2 Pharmacological methods of pain relief assessed as 'Very good' or 'Good' (NBT Survey 1990)

Method	Midwife		Woman		Partner		Midwives, women and partners	
	n	(%)	*n*	(%)	*n*	(%)	*n*	(%)
Entonox	4780	(85)	2956	(85)	2204	(84)	1332	(88)
Pethidine	3166	(84)	1468	(71)	1075	(72)	517	(58)
Epidural	1613	(91)	1043	(94)	772	(94)	512	(97)
Meptazinol	77	(75)	86	(84)	57	(75)	5	(50)
Diamorphine	108	(88)	99	(87)	88	(84)	17	(89)

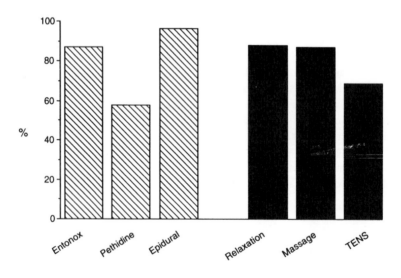

Fig. 8.1 The percentages of midwives, women and partners assessing various pharmacological and non-pharmacological methods as 'very good' or 'good' (NBT 1990).

> Gas and air was good at first for taking my mind off the pain but eventually just gave a high, causing confusion but no pain relief.

Pethidine was rated much higher by the midwife than by the woman or her partner.

> I had pethidine for the birth of my first baby, and felt relaxed and happy during the birth.
>
> Pethidine made me very drowsy. I feel that I may have been better equipped physically to push without it.
>
> I was very disappointed with the pethidine as I could not think straight and would not do as I was told. This was because the pethidine made me very sleepy.
>
> I asked for pethidine ... but I never did receive it. This was my second baby, I didn't enjoy the birth at all. My first baby I could have over again. I had a great labour as I received pethidine.
>
> Pethidine gave pain relief but brought labour to a standstill.

Perhaps the drowsiness of the woman following the administration of pethidine is associated with effective pain relief by the midwife. Despite the large numbers of adverse comments from the women, many will choose to use pethidine again in their next labour (see Ch. 5).

Epidural analgesia ranked as the most effective method in this study as in many others (Bundsen et al 1982, Morgan et al 1982, Avard & Nimrod 1985, Waldenström 1987). This technique prompted the most comments, not just on its effectiveness but also on the disappointment and distress caused when the promised epidural for which the couple had been prepared was not or could not be performed:

> There was only one anaesthetist in the maternity unit so my wife was told that she would have to wait at least an hour for an epidural, by which time it was too late.

Many couples commented that they had not been given sufficient information on epidurals; for example, the frequencies of top-ups, the need for intravenous fluids and the possibility of delays in siting the epidural. The majority gave very positive comments:

> Epidural improved both myself and my wife's enjoyment of the birth, by removing contraction pains completely and diminishing the stress and fatigue of the occasion.

Diamorphine was given in only 4% of labours but all these groups rated it highly when it was used.

Assessments were made not just by the midwife but also by the medical staff when they were present during the labour and therefore in a position to judge the effectiveness of the method used. These data have not been included in the comparison tables about non-pharmacological methods because the totals were too small apart from those referring to epidural (see Table 8.3).

In the majority of cases, methods other than epidural were rated as 'Poor' or 'No use' by this group. This may be because doctors only become involved in the care of labouring women when the pain relief method in use is inadequate and a request has now been made for a more powerful agent, e.g. epidural, or if the labour has been complicated by one or more factors resulting in an increased level of pain for the woman and subsequently a decrease in the level of effectiveness of the pain relief method she has been using.

FACTORS AFFECTING THE RELIEF OF PAIN AND ABILITY TO RELAX IN LABOUR

The women were asked, as an open question, to identify the factors which were most helpful and most unhelpful in relieving their pain in labour (Question 8 in Branch 2b). The answers were coded into 18 categories and can be seen in Tables 8.4 and

Table 8.3 The main methods of pain relief used recorded by the medical staff (NBT Survey 1990)

Method	Assessor	
	Obstetrician n	Anaesthetist n
Relaxation exercises	13	3
Massage	5	1
TENS	34	16
Pethidine	258	128
Entonox	332	173
Epidural	687	1239
General anaesthesia	260	256
Meptazinol	10	7
Diamorphine	43	27

Table 8.4 Pharmacological and non-pharmacological methods identified as helpful and unhelpful factors in the relief of pain (NBT Survey 1990)

Factor	Helpful		Unhelpful	
	n	(%)	n	(%)
Pethidine	750	(16.3)	374	(25.3)
Entonox	1837	(40.0)	565	(38.2)
Epidural	938	(20.4)	61	(4.1)
Other drugs	62	(1.3)	13	(0.9)
Relaxation exercises	765	(16.6)	302	(20.4)
TENS	86	(1.9)	79	(5.3)
Massage	162	(3.5)	86	(5.8)
TOTAL	4600		1480	

Table 8.5 Helpful and unhelpful factors in the relief of pain – other than pharmacological and non-pharmacological methods (NBT Survey 1990)

Factor	Helpful		Unhelpful	
	n	(%)	n	(%)
Companion	198	(34.5)	36	(7.5)
Choice – freedom/lack of	2	(0.3)	6	(1.2)
Bath/shower	46	(7.9)	11	(2.3)
Parentcraft classes	26	(4.5)	2	(0.4)
Advice – good/conflicting	1	(0.2)	7	(1.4)
Midwife/lack of Staff	93	(16.0)	30	(6.2)
Doctor	6	(1.0)	2	(0.4)
Position	36	(6.2)	160	(33.1)
Television/music	8	(1.4)	3	(0.6)
Bed	81	(14.0)	190	(39.4)
Mobility/immobility	84	(14.5)	36	(7.5)
TOTAL	581		483	

8.5 and in Figures 8.2 and 8.3. It will be noted that drugs and the alternative methods of pain relief comprise the majority of the answers with companion scoring next in the helpful column, and bed and position ranking high in the unhelpful column.

The methods of pain relief identified in this answer were cross-referenced with the methods actually used, and the percentages calculated (see Table 8.6 and Figure 8.2).

In every column the percentage of women who found the method to be helpful is higher than those who rated it unhelpful. In most cases it is twice as high, but not in relation to TENS where 22% found it helpful, 20% found it to be unhelpful. In the epidural category, 73% rated it as helpful and only 4% as unhelpful. If a ratio of helpful/unhelpful

Table 8.6 Methods of pain relief identified as helpful and unhelpful as a percentage of their use (NBT Survey 1990)

Factor	Helpful (%)	Unhelpful (%)
Relaxation exercises	32	13
Massage	22	12
TENS	22	20
Pethidine	28	14
Entonox	43	13
Epidural	73	4

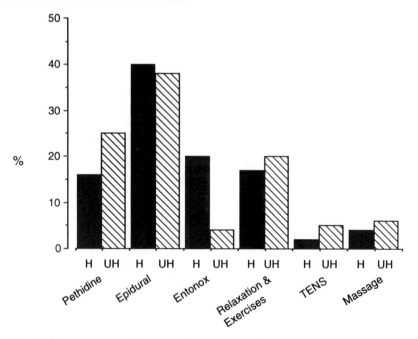

Fig. 8.2 The percentages of women using various methods of analgesia who found them to be helpful (H) or unhelpful (UH) (NBT 1990).

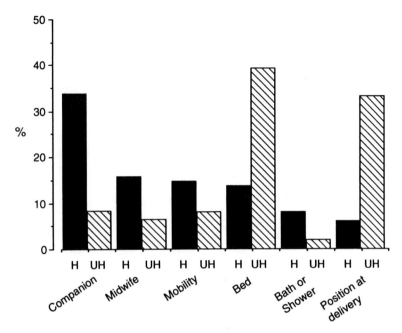

Fig. 8.3 The percentages of women reporting various non-analgesic factors influencing pain relief by helpful (H) and unhelpful (UH) (NBT 1990).

methods of analgesia were calculated among these women, epidural would be 18, Entonox 3 and pethidine 2 while relaxation would be 2, massage 2 and TENS 1. This may be considered a rough guide to the women's own opinion of pain relief.

Many gave comments relating to the factors which they had found helpful or not so helpful:

Companion:

> Most effective help towards pain relief during labour would appear to be from a supportive and caring partner and the midwifery staff.

Partner:

> The feelings of concern and elation have been tempered by a feeling of uselessness, almost to being in the way.

Classes:

> Information beforehand was invaluable. Gave confidence which was the best form of pain relief.

> I feel that the only way to relieve pain is to prepare the woman before she goes into labour. More emphasis should be put on the fact that giving birth to something that is 10 times the size of the orifice it's supposed to come out of will never be without pain.

Bed:

> Despite all the time and effort spent in antenatal class learning various positions, my wife spent most of her labour in bed. I feel that if she had been able to move around more freely her labour time may have been shortened.

> I feel that being completely stationary was unnecessary . . . being on my back I had no control over the pain.

> I was very happy that pain relief during labour was handled according to my wishes as expressed in the birth plan. I do, however, feel that I would have experienced considerably less pain had I not had to remain attached to the monitor throughout virtually the whole process.

Television:

> England scoring against Belgium was a great help (comment from a partner – the study was done in the midst of the World Cup in Association Football).

Questions 9 and 10 had asked the woman if she had been able to relax and, if not, what had interfered with this process. Table 8.7 and Figure 8.4 show a breakdown of the answers.

Anxiety was identified as by far the biggest problem but the women could give more than one answer to this question; for example, she may have ticked 'anxiety' but also 'restricted to bed by the fetal monitor'. Further examination showed that 710 women out of the 1193 (60%) had ticked anxiety only. More primigravidae than multi-gravidae highlighted anxiety as an interfering factor as did women who had had more than one midwife providing their care.

The size of the unit in which these women delivered their babies was considered to determine whether that could be an influencing factor on the women expressing anxiety. The four sizes of units, categorised according to the number of births per annum, were examined in each region and Table 8.8 shows the results.

A wide variation can be seen in the small and medium units throughout the regions. In the small units, the range of percentage of women identifying anxiety is 0–39% and in the medium units the range is 0–26%. In the large and very large units, however, the range is much narrower, 14–27% in the large units and 13–25% in the very large units, with means of 19% and 18%, respectively.

Table 8.7 Number of women who were able to relax in labour and factors which interfered with this process. Some women gave more than one answer so data are not correlative (NBT Survey 1990)

	n	(%)[a]
Were you able to relax?		
Yes	4323	(74.5)
No	3072	(25.5)
If no, what interfered?		
Restricted to bed	629	(9.7)
Unfamiliar surroundings	204	(3.1)
Strangers	93	(1.4)
Noise	80	(1.2)
Monitor	430	(6.6)
Bright lights	47	(0.7)
Too many people	73	(1.1)
Conflicting advice	107	(1.6)
Anxiety	1193	(18.4)
Other	216	(3.3)

[a]Percentage of total survey population.

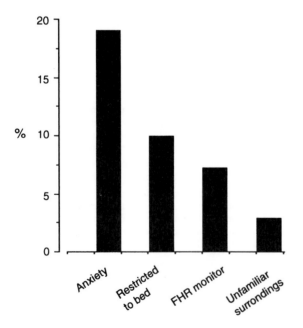

Fig. 8.4 The percentages of women who, having reported they were not able to relax, identified what interfered with that relaxation (NBT 1990).

Table 8.8 Proportion of women who identified anxiety as a restricting factor according to size of unit (NBT Survey 1990)

Region	Size of units			
	Small <500 (%)	Medium 500–2000 (%)	Large 2001–4000 (%)	Very large >4000 (%)
Northern	0	13	26	22
Yorkshire	0	16	18	14
Trent	28	11	18	18
East Anglia	0	8	18	13
North West Thames	14	14	19	13
North East Thames	0	23	18	0
South East Thames	0	9	14	0
South West Thames	0	23	22	25
Wessex	0	24	19	17
Oxford	0	0	18	17
South Western	20	18	17	25
West Midlands	4	6	17	16
Mersey	0	26	27	23
North Western	20	21	21	18
Channel Islands	0	8	0	0
Northern Ireland	0	13	19	0
Scotland	39	18	21	15
Wales	10	18	23	22
Armed Services	11	21	0	0
Independent	8	0	0	0
TOTAL	10	15	19	18

Cross-tabulations of women reporting anxiety by the methods they had planned to use and actually used were carried out (see Table 8.9 and Fig. 8.5).

The results show significant differences. The first are those relating to the women who used some form of pain relief although they had planned to use none:

> My labour was so different from my expectations that my preconceived intentions regarding pain relief became irrelevant.
>
> I was disappointed with my ability to cope with pain; perhaps I had unrealistic expectations.

The second set of columns relates to the group of women who planned to have an epidural but actually did not get one. No matter what method they used in place of the epidural, this group had the highest score as regards anxiety expressed. This was reflected in comments from both the women and partners:

> There appears to be a certain reluctance among midwives to give epidurals.
>
> To be told that staff shortages meant that there was no-one around to give me my epidural upset and panicked me. I do realise the NHS has problems but it is wrong to hand out books promising pain relief options that are not available in practice.

THE TEENAGE AND THE OLDER PRIMIGRAVID GROUPS

Maternal age is an important factor in the outcome of pregnancy since higher rates of complications occur at the age extremes – under 20 years and 35 years and over. The problems of the teenager relate

Table 8.9 Number of women identifying anxiety compared to methods planned and used (NBT Survey 1990)

Pain relief method	Planned and used (%)	Planned but not used (%)
Relaxation exercises	17	20
Massage	20	18
TENS	19	15
Entonox	20	17
Pethidine	21	20
Epidural	15	24
No method	6	18

to the fact that she is not yet fully mature and often cannot adapt physically to the pregnancy. Antenatal care may be less then ideal due to concealment of the pregnancy or to lack of interest to attend either the antenatal clinic or the parentcraft classes. The older primigravida has special problems related to the progression of disorders associated with increasing age such as hypertensive disease or diabetes. She is more prone to chromosomal disorders and multiple pregnancies and there is an increased possibility of intrauterine growth retardation. The perinatal mortality rates are highest in this group.

Knowing the woman's age at the beginning of pregnancy is central to planning her care, yet in 14% of the questionnaires in this study maternal age was not recorded, a significant deficiency. Perhaps the midwives omitted this information believing that it was irrelevant to our study although the specific question had been asked or maybe it was omitted because it was not known. If the latter applied we are failing in providing individualised care according to the women's needs. False modesty about a woman's age should stay in the drawing room and not enter the antenatal clinics or classes.

There were 722 women under 20 years old (7.0%), a little lower proportion than national data (8.1%). Of these, 359 completed their questionnaires at the time of the baby's birth and 33 of these were included in the follow-up survey at 6 weeks after the birth. Only 18 women in this group were of Asian origin (2.5% vs. 4.7% in all age groups). The majority (80%) were nulliparae and over twice as many (9.5%) were unsupported than the 4.3% in the total study population. There was a higher incidence of spontaneous vertex deliveries and a lower incidence of Caesarean sections than the total population – 7.5% vs. 11.4%. This figure is similar to those of the North West Thames study where 7.3% of the teenage group had Caesarean sections (Paterson et al 1991).

At the other end of the reproductive range, 704 women (6.8%) in the study were aged 35 years and over; this compares with 8.5% in England and Wales in 1989. All ethnic groups were represented proportionately and there was no significant difference in the presence of social support. Fewer women in this group delivered their babies spontaneously – 74.9% compared to 78.9% in all age groups. A higher proportion required a Caesarean

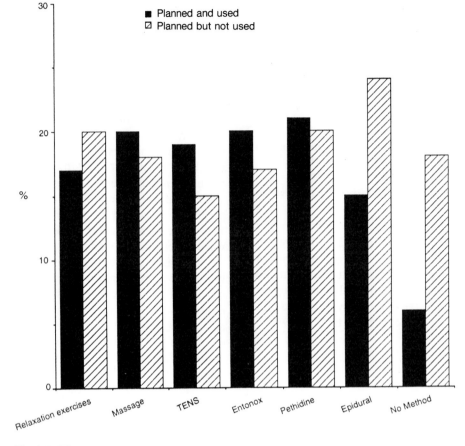

Fig. 8.5   The percentages of women identifying anxiety, comparing the method of analgesia planned and used with those who had a method planned but did not use it (NBT 1990).

section – 15.9% vs. 11.4% in all age groups. In the North West Thames study, 18.9% of women aged 35 and over had Caesarean sections (Paterson et al 1991).

The main methods of pain relief used by both groups are shown in Table 8.10. Comparisons can be made not only between the two age groups but also between each group and the total survey population. It can be noted that pethidine is much more commonly used by the teenage group than by the others, while transcutaneous electrical nerve stimulation (TENS) is the least popular. TENS may have been a less well known method in this group, for only 37% attended parentcraft classes compared with 53.6% in the older primigravidae group.

In Table 8.11 the methods of pain relief which the women would choose for their next labour are shown. This information was drawn from the

follow-up survey, hence the smaller numbers. As in Table 8.10, Entonox is the most popular method in all groups, with pethidine again a popular choice in the teenage group and TENS in the older primigravidae group.

Among the 33 teenagers who were included in the follow-up study, 29 said that they were feeling physically well 6 weeks after the delivery but four women were depressed and two of these said that they did not feel confident in caring for their babies. One woman, 18 years old, commented:

> I wish people in the hospital had told me more. My boyfriend was more helpful than the staff when I was in pain.

The over 35 year old group compared well with the total survey population as regards physical health 6

Table 8.10 Methods of pain relief used as identified by the women in Branch 2B (NBT Survey 1990)

Group	Relaxation n	(%)	Massage n	(%)	TENS n	(%)	Entonox n	(%)	Pethidine n	(%)	Epidural n	(%)
Teenagers (n = 721)	40	(5.5)	72	(9.9)	16	(2.2)	510	(70)	386	(53)	128	(17)
Primigravidae 35 + (n = 704)	43	(6.2)	50	(7.3)	45	(6.5)	412	(60)	204	(28)	99	(14)
Total respondents (n = 6093)	2073	(3.4)	1178	(19.3)	335	(5.5)	3665	(60)	2247	(36.9)	1178	(19.3)

Table 8.11 Methods of choice next time – follow-up survey (NBT Survey 1990)

Group	Relaxation n	(%)	Massage n	(%)	TENS n	(%)	Entonox n	(%)	Pethidine n	(%)	Epidural n	(%)
Teenagers (n = 33)	16	(48)	11	(33)	2	(6)	26	(78)	18	(54)	8	(24)
Primigravidae 35 + (n = 88)	65	(74)	26	(29)	14	(16)	62	(70)	26	(29)	21	(24)
Total respondents (n = 1149)	738	(64)	412	(36)	157	(13)	751	(65)	458	(40)	315	(27)

weeks after the delivery; 88 answered questions and fewer, however, felt very happy or very confident at handling their babies – 32% vs. 37% and 15% vs. 21%, respectively.

HOME CONFINEMENTS

All women who gave birth during the week of the survey were invited to participate irrespective of the place of confinement. The dissemination of the study information and questionnaire to individual community and independent midwives and the coordination of the data collection had been done by the Head of Midwifery Services within each maternity unit. This was both complex and time-consuming for the Coordinator; this may be the reason that two-thirds of the expected number of home confinements were missing from the study.

In the survey week, 48 women (0.47% of total) filled in questionnaires having delivered their babies at home; there was also one woman who gave birth unexpectedly in the antenatal ward of the maternity unit. From national data one would have expected about 1% (about 140) of deliveries to have been at home, with about half of these being planned. Of the 48 home confinements, 32 were planned, a higher than average proportion than that usually recorded – about 55% accidental and 45% planned. In this group, 29 women and 26 partners returned their questionnaires and 13 were included

in the follow-up survey. Among the unplanned group, nine women and nine partners returned their questionnaires and three were also included in the follow-up.

There were no women of Afro-Caribbean origin in either group. Amongst the planned group, 14 were aged 30 years and over vs. 5 in the unplanned group. There was no significant difference between the groups either in marital status or support. Ten of the planned group and four of those who had unplanned home births were from social classes I and II; 22 of the former were multiparae and there were no preterm labours, whereas 14 out of 17 of those who had not planned were multiparae and three babies in this group were born before the 37th completed week of gestation (i.e. they had preterm labours). None of the differences are significant and the figures are too small to use percentages.

One woman who laboured at home as planned had to be transferred to hospital for forceps delivery with epidural analgesia for delay in the first stage of labour. Two other women with planned home deliveries had to be admitted to hospital for manual removal of placenta. Hence the in-labour transfer rate among reported planned home deliveries was 3/32.

All babies were born alive with 96% of the planned group having an Apgar score of 8 or more at 5 minutes after birth vs. 84% of the unplanned group.

Table 8.12 shows the methods of pain relief used by women who delivered at home.

Seven of the 29 women in the booked group said they had attended NCT classes in preparation for parenthood, i.e. 24% vs 5.3% of the total survey population. Four had attended parentcraft classes held at the hospital, and four at the health centre.

28 women booked for home confinement said they had been able to relax in labour vs. 5 of 9 in the unplanned group. In 89% of the former group, the partner had been present all through the labour, and in 86% continuity of care had been achieved by one midwife throughout the labour. Women in this group reported that the presence of a companion and the use of relaxation exercises had been the main factors in helping them relax. Only one woman identified anxiety as a factor which interfered with her ability to relax.

I believe I had a natural delivery because I was at home and was attended by two midwives I trusted. My labour took quite a jump after my waters broke suddenly ... if I had had to go to hospital at that point I know I would have accepted pain relief.

In their choice of methods of pain relief for their next labour, no-one would choose pethidine but only one woman had experience of it on this occasion. We do not know from this survey if they had used pethidine at other previous deliveries. The majority of these women would choose relaxation exercises, massage and Entonox 'because they worked well for this labour'. One woman wanted to

try epidural next time even though she would still choose to have the next baby at home.

Of the 13 women booked for homebirths who were included in the follow-up survey 6 weeks after the birth, 11 said they had enjoyed it; 12 were satisfied with the care they had received from their midwives, and 6 out of 10 were satisfied with the pain relief (three women omitted to answer this question).

The difference in pain quality between home and hospital was staggering. The pain was more intense flat on my back in hospital than at any stage at home.

One woman had now decided that she would choose pethidine after all, while two would now prefer to use no form of analgesia.

All the women in the booked group would choose to have their next baby at home. Two of the three women who had an unplanned delivery at home would choose to have their next baby there now.

STILLBIRTHS

There were 52 mothers who had stillbirths in the study, i.e. 5/1000, which is comparable with the present national rate of 4.7 per 1000 total births. 23 women in this group completed their sections of the questionnaire as did 18 of their partners.

There were no women of Afro-Caribbean origin in the group, but there was a higher number of women of Asian origin – 11.5% vs. 4.8% in the total survey population. The age of the mother was not significantly different from the total group. There was a higher proportion of separated women but no difference in relation to the support they had in this pregnancy; 28 women were nulliparae (53.8%) and a higher proportion came from social class V and unemployed categories.

The number of stillbirths per region can be seen in Table 8.13. Eight of the 52 cases had experienced an antepartum haemorrhage in this pregnancy and three had had investigations for fetal growth retardation. There were three sets of twins. 21 babies were preterm and 17 were of low birth weight (eight weights were not recorded). One woman used no form of pain relief. The most

Table 8.12 Methods of pain relief used by the women who delivered at home; some women used more than one method (NBT Survey 1990)

Method	Planned[a]	Unplanned[b]
None	7	3
Relaxation exercises	8	3
Massage	13	1
TENS	1	2
Acupuncture	1	0
Homeopathy	5	0
Entonox	12	5
Pethidine	1	0
Meptazinol	1	0
TOTAL	49	14

[a]Number of planned home deliveries by method used.
[b]Number of unplanned home deliveries by method used.

Table 8.13 Number of stillbirths reported during the study, by Region (NBT Survey 1990)

Region	SB[a]	Q[b]	Rate[c]
Northern	1	346	2.8
Yorkshire	0	700	0
Trent	4	911	4.4
East Anglia	3	476	6.3
North West Thames	3	633	4.7
North East Thames	4	613	6.5
South East Thames	1	518	1.9
South West Thames	3	478	6.2
Wessex	5	404	12.0
Oxford	2	507	4.0
South Western	10	535	18.0
West Midlands	1	959	1.0
Mersey	3	325	9.0
North Western	3	793	3.0
Channel Islands	0	37	0
Northern Ireland	2	437	4.5
Scotland	6	1 051	5.7
Wales	1	497	2.0
Armed Services	0	54	0
Independent	0	42	0
TOTAL	52	10 316	5.0

[a]Number of stillbirths.
[b]Number of questionnaires completed.
[c]Stillbirths per 1000 recorded births.

common methods used were Entonox and pethidine – 11 women of the 23 – while only four had an epidural.

None of these women nor their partners made any comments on the pain nor on the methods of pain relief they had used. Perhaps this illustrates that pain is not as significant a feature of the labour and delivery as it is in the case of the birth of a live baby.

One woman commented:

> I had twins 6 weeks prematurely and one was stillborn. I feel unhappy that I was asked if I wanted to see him while I was still coming round from the operation. At that time I was in no state to make such a decision and said 'No' because I was afraid of how I would react. I very much regret this and feel I should have been given time to discuss it with my husband.

No data were collected on babies born during the week of the survey who later died in the first week of life, therefore a perinatal mortality rate cannot be calculated. Three women, however, took part in the follow-up survey despite the fact that their babies had died.

PERINEAL DAMAGE AND REPAIR

The discomfort and distress suffered by women as a result of perineal damage and repair was highlighted by both the women and their partners in their open comments in this survey. Although most of the questionnaire was aimed at obtaining information about pain in labour and the factors which may affect this the survey did ask questions on perineal pain. No data were gathered in this survey on the degree of perineal damage, the status of the person who inserted the sutures or the length of time which elapsed between the delivery of the baby and the repair of the perineum. This is separate research which is being carried out elsewhere at the moment.

> There was one and a half hour's gap between giving birth and having stitches. When eventually done, they proved much more of a problem as far as pain goes than anything that happened during labour. It seems to me that more needs to be done to ensure stitching is pain free and promptly done.

Question 18 in the women's questionnaire in Branch 2 asked her if she had stitches and what form of pain relief was used. Question 19 in the follow-up survey in Branch 3 asked the woman 6 weeks after the birth of her baby if she was suffering from any perineal discomfort. 3757 women out of 5241 who answered Question 18 said they had perineal sutures for either a tear or an episiotomy; 64% of women who had a spontaneous vaginal delivery had sutures as did 98% who had an operative vaginal delivery. Methods of pain relief used for the actual repair of the perineum are listed in Table 8.14 and shown in Figure 8.6.

Only about 7% had no analgesia and almost 90% had anaesthesia of some form.

Table 8.15 and Figure 8.7 show the relationship between method of delivery and perineal discomfort

Table 8.14 Methods of pain relief used for perineal repair (NBT Survey 1990)

Methods	n	(%)
Local anaesthesia	1758	(45.2)
Nitrous oxide/oxygen	1215	(31.2)
Epidural	526	(13.5)
None	266	(6.8)
Don't know	126	(3.2)

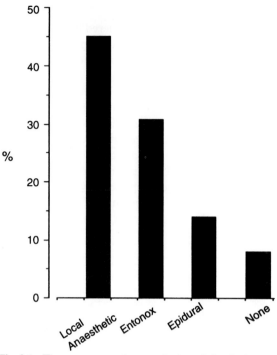

Fig. 8.6 The percentages of women having stitches in the perineal area by the anaesthetic or analgesic methods used (NBT 1990).

Table 8.15 Method of delivery by perineal discomfort (NBT Survey 1990)

Method of delivery	Perineal discomfort					
	A lot		A little		None	
	n	(%)	n	(%)	n	(%)
Spontaneous	148	(19)	351	(46)	269	(35)
Operative vaginal	48	(54)	32	(39)	6	(7)

6 weeks after the birth of the baby. According to Sleep et al (1984), 23% of women report some degree of discomfort 10 days following a normal delivery. In this study, 46% of the women who took part in the follow-up survey stated that they were still experiencing a little perineal discomfort while 19% reported that they were suffering a lot 6 weeks later. This group all had spontaneous vertex deliveries. Only 7% in the group who had operative vaginal deliveries stated they had no perineal discomfort 6 weeks after the birth of their baby.

Women by this time are no longer receiving care from their community midwives. They therefore need to have the courage and ability to make the effort to visit the general practitioner early or to

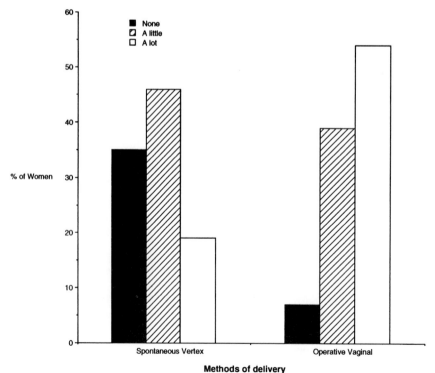

Fig 8.7 Method of delivery by perineal discomfort – see text (NBT 1990).

endure the problem until the postnatal appointment date. Generally those following spontaneous delivery had less discomfort than those who had an operative vaginal birth. In the follow-up survey, women were asked to describe how they had been feeling emotionally since the birth. Table 8.16 shows a breakdown of their answers.

Relationships between emotional state and perineal discomfort were investigated and can be seen in Table 8.17 and Figure 8.8. While 21% of happy women still reported a lot of perineal pain, 40% of depressed women did. Some 88% of the follow-up group of women were not depressed and 80% of these had no pain or only a little. This relationship is not necessarily evidence of cause and effect; depressed women may well feel more pain from a perineal wound than a non-depressed woman would feel from a similar wound.

It is clear that women are unprepared for the pain they suffered both during the process of perineal repair and during the healing stages in the postnatal period. They found this unnecessary and less acceptable compared to the pain of labour, which they understand as being a natural means to an end.

Table 8.16 Emotional state 6 weeks after birth (NBT Survey 1990)

Emotional state	n	(%)
Very happy	423	(37)
Happy	585	(51.1)
Quite depressed	72	(6.3)
Very depressed	17	(1.5)
Other	44	(3.8)
Don't know	3	(0.3)
TOTAL	1144	(100.0)

Table 8.17 Perineal discomfort by emotional state (NBT Survey 1990)

Emotional state	Perineal discomfort					
	A lot		A little		None	
	n	(%)	n	(%)	n	(%)
Happy	191	(21.5)	398	(45)	297	(33.5)
Depressed	30	(40.5)	27	(36.5)	17	(23)

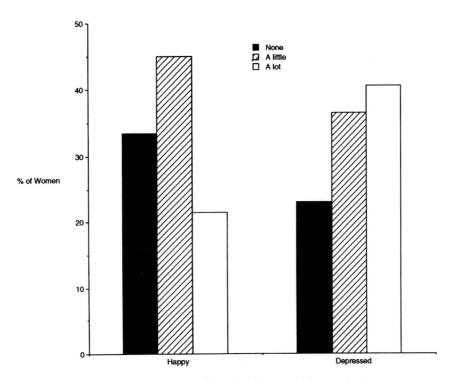

Fig 8.8 The percentages of women reporting perineal discomfort by emotional state – see text (NBT 1990).

> I wish I could have been completely numb for the stitches, as they are the overriding memory of the whole birth and did in fact spoil what had been a painful but special experience.

Professionals are all aware of the implications of perineal damage and repair to the woman as she recovers from childbirth and is coping with the physical and emotional changes as well as caring for her newborn baby.

A perineal suturing trial, funded by the National Birthday Trust, is now in progress at the Ipswich Hospital. This will compare the effects of skin apposition to skin sutures to determine whether a substantial part of the discomfort is caused by the actual sutures to the skin rather than the deeper layers. The findings from this study may enable us to improve the care of women after delivery and reduce the incidence of perineal discomfort in the puerperium. In general, such research is seen as unglamorous and it is more difficult to obtain funding for it than for research apparently directed at saving lives. However, it is clear from our survey that such work is badly needed, and would be welcomed by many women. Equally, it is unlikely that having a baby can ever be made a painless process, and so women must be educated that perineal discomfort or even pain cannot always be avoided and for some is an inescapable part of becoming a mother.

REFERENCES

Avard D M, Nimrod C M 1985 Risks and benefits of an obstetrical epidural service. Birth 12: 215–225
Bundsen P et al 1982 Pain relief during delivery. Acta Obstetrica Gynaecologica Scandinavica 61: 289–297
Morgan B M et al 1982 Analgesia and satisfaction in childbirth. Lancet ii: 808–810
Paterson C M et al 1991 Evaluating the maternity services. British Journal of Obstetrics and Gynaecology 98: 1073–1078
Savage W 1986 A Savage enquiry. Virago Press, London
Sleep J, Grant A 1984 West Berkshire Perineal Management Trial British Medical Journal 295: 749–51
Waldenström U 1988 Midwives' attitudes to pain relief during labour and delivery. Midwifery 4: 48–57

9. The effects of pain relief on the baby

H. Gamsu

THE POPULATION

There were 10 300 live births included in this study, born in 293 different units in the UK and at home. The population seems to have been a healthy one, if one compares the low birth weight rate (5.9%) in this study population with that of England and Wales in 1990 (6.8%). Only 6.5% of cases were admitted to a neonatal unit indicating a low risk population with a low admission rate. The Caesarean section rate was 11.4% and that of assisted delivery 9.9%, both a little lower than the national average indicating a higher percentage of normal women without problems in the survey than in the general population. So we may expect it to be for the babies.

PAIN RELIEF USED

Most methods of analgesia were available in the obstetric units, pethidine and Entonox being available in more than 99% of hospitals and epidural anaesthesia in only 73%. Alternative methods were only available in 10% but relaxation methods were used in 92% of these hospitals.

One or more methods of analgesia were used in 61% of women, whereas in greater than 30% there was no report of analgesia having been used. Entonox, available in 99% of the units, was used by 60% of the women. Pethidine, available in 98%, was given to 38% of the women. Epidural, although reported to be available in 73% of the units, was only given to 18% of the women, and general anaesthesia to 7.9% of the total. Other drugs (meptazinol, diamorphine, lignocaine and a few others) were given to 15% of the mothers; other methods such as relaxation etc. were used in 17.3%.

EFFECTS OF ANALGESIC AGENTS ON THE FETUS

Most drugs when given to the mother are transferred to the fetus. The amount that passes, the concentration reached and that which is maintained in fetal tissues depends upon a number of maternal and fetal factors. The surface area of the placenta, the degree of placental binding of the drug and uterine blood flow as well as the characteristics of the drugs themselves such as their molecular size and shape, their degree of ionisation, their lipid solubility, and the degree they are protein bound are all factors which influence the levels and the effects of drugs in the fetus. Non-protein bound and non-ionised drugs are freely diffusable. Basic drugs will tend to concentrate in the fetus in whom the pH is lower than that of the mother.

In the fetus, blood levels of any transmitted drug will fall progressively in a cranial direction as the umbilical venous blood becomes progressively diluted by admixture of blood from other vessels, but since there is normally both a high cerebral blood flow and the blood-brain barrier in the fetus is poorly developed, distribution of drugs to the brain is disproportionately higher.

If the fetus is chronically hypoxic, the brain is likely to receive an even greater blood flow associated with the expected redistribution of blood in this state, which is accompanied by decreased blood flow in the descending aorta and increased flow to the upper part of the body. The heart muscle itself receives a higher concentration of administered drugs in these cirumstances. In the hypoxic fetus, worsening acidosis will increase ionisation and lead to increased fetal drug retention and decreased transfer of drugs and their metabolites back to the mother.

A number of other mechanisms will also influence the effect of drugs on the fetus, including maternal hypotension which reduces placental blood flow and so leads to fetal hypoxia. Maternal hypoxia is especially likely to result from complications associated with general anaesthesia or drugs causing respiratory depression in the mother. Hypoventilation in the mother giving rise to hypercapnia may predispose to fetal hypoxia because of reduced placental perfusion following placental bed vasoconstriction. Respiratory alkalosis from maternal hyperventilation also causes a shift in the oxygen dissociation curve to the left, thus causing less release of oxygen from maternal to fetal haemoglobin.

Aortocaval compression, a notorious cause of decreased uterine perfusion if the woman is in the supine position, is accompanied by diminished venous return and hence diminished cardiac output. The unanaesthetised mother can compensate for this to some extent by an increase in heart rate and peripheral vascular resistance, but the deeply anaesthetised woman or one who has had an epidural or spinal anaesthetic must be watched carefully and nursed in a lateral tilt position as these compensatory mechanisms may not be possible. (For further reading, see Albin 1987).

EFFECTS OF ANALGESICS ON THE NEWBORN

After birth, analgesic and anaesthetic agents are prone to delay the onset of breathing in the newborn; they influence the Apgar score and cause lower PaO_2 and raised $PaCO_2$ levels. With some agents, depression may continue and result in a decreased respiratory rate, reduced tidal volume and hence a lowered minute volume. The baby is more likely to be hypotonic and sleepy. Visual alertness might be decreased and the baby is likely to be disinterested in feeding. Sucking frequency and sucking pressure are reduced.

Subtle effects of these drugs might be the result of both maternal and neonatal depression. For example, eye to eye contact and mothering behaviour might be influenced by them. Effects on the baby of maternally administered analgesics may still be detectable hours, days and possibly even weeks after

birth with documented diminished alertness, reduced muscle tone and alterations of behaviour and motor function (Belsey et al 1981). A constellation of signs has been assembled into various neurobehavioural scores which seek to classify the behaviour of the newborn. These tests have been described by Brazelton (1973), Scanlon (1974) and Amiel-Tison (1982). All these neurobehavioural scales assess the response of the baby to visual, auditory and sensory stimuli and attempt to quantitate alertness and other items such as the baby's consolability, irritability, activity, the presence of abnormal movements and other abnormal neurological signs. Babies exposed to maternally administered analgesic drugs are known to generate lower scores using these tests than do those of the controls.

There have been suggestions that there are longer-lasting effects of maternally administered analgesics. Broman & Brackbill (1978), using data from the Collaborative Perinatal Project, suggest that there was lower development of motor skills and cognitive ability up to the age of 7 years but the selection of the group they studied might have been faulty and there was no control group. In fact, Ounstead et al (1980, 1981) have reported no long-term effect of from obstetric analgesia and anaesthesia at the age of 4 years. This also included lack of effect of general and epidural anaesthesia.

THE EFFECT OF SPECIFIC ANALGESIC AGENTS

Entonox

This mixture of nitrous oxide with oxygen is unlikely to cause neonatal depression, even though placental transfer of nitrous oxide is rapid. The concentration of nitrous oxide reached in the fetus is low and elimination is rapid. Maternal hyperventilation to achieve adequate inhalation analgesia could lead to reduced fetal oxygenation by causing constriction of uteroplacental vessels. Reduced perfusion of the intervillus space and the resulting alkalosis might, by shifting the oxygen dissociation curve to the left, lead to impaired release of maternal oxygen to the fetus. Little effect has been shown on the neurobehavioural score of babies at 2 and 24 hours.

Pethidine

Virginia Apgar and colleagues were among the first to demonstrate free transfer of pethidine across the human placenta (Apgar et al 1952); this is greater after intravenous than after intramuscular administration and the peak levels are higher. This narcotic agent is poorly protein bound in the fetus and newborn and highly ionised, acidosis increasing this ionisation. The elimination half-life of pethidine in the baby is long, about 18–23 hours compared to up to 5 hours in the mother. 95% of pethidine is excreted in 2–3 days but the total elimination time is 2–3 times that of the mother. Nor-pethidine, one of the major metabolites of the drug, has an even longer elimination half-life and is also a potent respiratory depressant. Also it is less effectively antagonised by naloxone.

The effect of pethidine therefore depends on the dose, the injection to delivery interval, the route of injection, the timing of injection and whether the injections are repeated.

> I did not realise that injections are not given in later stages of labour because of their effect on the baby. If I had known this I would have asked for an epidural or other injection earlier.
>
> This time my labour was short and although I asked for pethidine the midwife advised against it as the baby was coming quickly and the drug would make her sleepy. I am glad I did not have any.

Naloxone

If this narcotic antagonist is administered intravenously the effect of narcotic agents is reversed for a few hours but at 4 and 24 hours neonatal behaviour and feeding behaviour are still depressed (Wiener et al 1977). Naloxone 200 µg i.m. given to the baby soon after birth has been shown to result in more sustained improvement in neonatal respiration, feeding, habituation to sound, and alertness.

> I would have liked to have known that pethidine could have been given in doses from 50–150 mg and that the baby could have had an antidote to pethidine after birth.

EPIDURAL ANAESTHESIA

All commonly used local anaesthetics cross the placenta readily and may affect the fetus. They are of low molecular weight and are lipid soluble. Lignocaine is particularly likely to cause side-effects, whereas bupivacaine, which is more protein bound, is less likely to be transferred. The fetal, and hence neonatal consequences of maternal hypotension are more likely if preloading of the mother with fluid has been omitted and if she is lying supine. Lignocaine has been found to affect neonatal behaviour adversely soon after birth, but most of these effects become insignificant after 24 hours. Epidural anaesthesia has been associated with fewer babies with depressed Apgar scores than is likely to occur after general anaesthesia.

> I would have chosen an epidural but was unsure of the effect on the baby, which I wanted to be minimal.

Early neonatal neurobehaviour has been found to be little affected by epidural bupivacaine but there is some evidence of an effect on the Brazelton neonatal behavioural assessment score; there is a decrement in attention and responsiveness at first but with increased muscle tone some days after birth (Belsey et al 1981); Wiener et al (1979) showed reduced muscle tone for up to 48 hours after birth.

GENERAL ANAESTHESIA

Neurobehavioural effects have been shown to occur after induction agents have been administered. These effects are dose dependent and the early neonatal neurobehavioural score may be lower in the first 48 hours as a result of these agents. An induction to delivery interval greater than 30 minutes is associated with more pronounced effects so the time the woman has a general anaesthetic before delivery should not be prolonged; many anaesthetists await the arrival of the scrubbed surgeon at the table side before starting their induction although there is no evidence that a short delay from induction to delivery is harmful. Hypoxia and hypotension during general anaesthesia are both likely to lead to fetal and neonatal complications. The Apgar score at 1 and 5 minutes is lower and the need for intermittent positive pressure ventilation (IPPV) of the newborn is greater with general anaesthesia than with epidural anaesthesia.

CONDITION OF THE BABY AT BIRTH

Apgar scores

In the National Birthday Trust survey, 2.5% of those who reported had a baby with a 1–minute Apgar score of less than 4, and 11% scores of 4–6 at 1 minute. At 5 minutes 0.4% had scores of less than 4 and 1.5% scores of 4–6; 0.5% of the newborn babies had scores of less than 7 at 10 minutes.

Table 9.1 and Figure 9.1 show that, compared with babies whose mothers had no analgesia, Entonox analgesia seemed not to be associated with a much higher rate of low Apgar scores at either 1 or 5 minutes and these two groups of babies thus behaved similarly. In contrast, there was a striking association between low scores at both 1 and 5 minutes with general anaesthesia and an association with diamorphine, meptazinol and to a lesser extent pethidine, but only minimally with epidural anaesthesia. The differential effect is seen more closely in Figure 9.1 for here are plotted those babies whose mothers had a single method of analgesia only, thus avoiding any compound effects. The fact that lower Apgar scores were more likely to be encountered with Caesarean section was not surprising. A similar association was seen with operative vaginal delivery (Table 9.2).

Table 9.1 Numbers and percentages of babies with an Apgar score less than 7 by pain relief given (NBT Survey 1990)

Pain relief	1 min		5 min	
	n	(%)	*n*	(%)
None	25	(7.5)	3	(1.0)
Entonox only	180	(9.1)	23	(1.2)
Entonox plus other	841	(13.0)	112	(1.7)
Pethidine only	77	(12.3)	8	(1.3)
Pethidine plus other	618	(15.5)	82	(2.1)
Epidural only	90	(10.5)	14	(1.6)
Epidural plus other	337	(15.0)	40	(1.9)
GA only	109	(29.8)	29	(8.0)
GA plus other	264	(34.2)	59	(7.7)
Diamorphine	8	(19.0)	1	(2.3)
Diamorphine plus other	81	(19.3)	12	(3.3)
Meptazinol only	11	(16.2)	1	(1.4)
Meptazinol plus other	39	(11.3)	3	(9.0)

Table 9.2 Percentages of babies with Apgar score less than 7 by method of delivery (NBT Survey 1990)

Method of Delivery	<7 at 1 min		<7 at 5 min	
	n	(%)	n	(%)
Spontaneous	811	(11.1)	95	(1.3)
Operative vaginal	186	(19.3)	23	2.4
Caesarean section	296	(27.5)	16	(4.0)
TOTAL	1293		134	

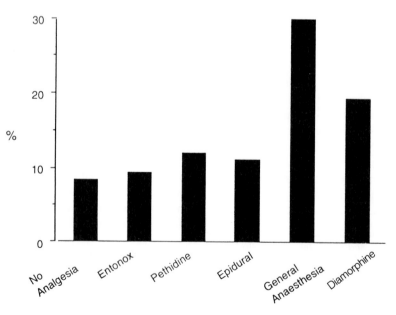

Fig. 9.1 The percentages of babies with an Apgar score of less than 7 at 1 minute by the method of analgesia (NBT Survey 1990).

This effect is compounded by the high proportion of babies delivered by Caesarean section who were of low birth weight. Since some of these Caesarean sections would be preceded by fetal distress and would thus have been performed as an emergency, the degree of the low Apgar scores caused by the general anaesthetic could not be apportioned. The likelihood that general anaesthesia would have been used for Caesarean section for delivery of mothers of low gestation and babies with low birthweight can be seen in the accompanying Table 9.3.

TIME OF ONSET OF SPONTANEOUS BREATHING

These data were recorded in 16.4%. Of these, 70.5% breathed spontaneously within 1 minute and 99% within 10 minutes. 11.5% of babies whose mothers were given Entonox breathed only after 3 minutes and a similar percentage breathed spontaneously after maternal pethidine administration (10%) and epidural (12.3%), whereas for the reasons already outlined the onset of spontaneous breathing was delayed in a greater percentage (23.4%) of those babies delivered after general anaesthesia.

RESUSCITATION

About 30% of babies received some assistance with breathing at birth; 73% had facial oxygen (20% of the total population), 30.8% bag and mask ventilation (8.5% of the total), and 11% intubation (3.0% of the total). Of those needing ventilation, in 2.4% this was done within 3 minutes of being born; in 92% assisted ventilation ceased within 10 minutes.

Resuscitation was performed by a midwife in 56% of instances, by a paediatrician in 55% and other staff in 2.5% of cases. Naloxone was given to only 7.2% of all babies (in 87% of cases by the intramuscular route) yet opiate drugs had been given to over 45% and pethidine to 40% of mothers. 63% of the babies with an Apgar score of less than 7 at 1 minute received naloxone.

Over 80% of mothers given pethidine received 200 mg or less; 73% of these were in the first stage of labour, with 60% in the middle or late part of that first stage. Table 9.4 and Figure 9.2 show the requirements for babies whose mothers were given single analgesic agents. Entonox alone given to the mother resulted in less need for oxygen and IPPV but the need for oxygen and IPPV was greatest in those babies delivered by Caesarean section, particularly if general anaesthesia was used.

EARLY EXAMINATION OF THE BABY

The survey reported that about 70% of all babies were examined, three-quarters of them by paediatric staff (65% by the paediatric SHO). In 19.3% examination was performed by the midwife and in 10.1% by either an obstetrician or the general practitioner. Over 75% of these examinations were performed in the first 24 hours.

A number of conditions were reported overall but only a small proportion of those (0.5%) were noted by the first examiner as many arose later. Hypotonia and excessive sleepiness were noted in 1.2%. Hypoglycaemia, hypothermia and apnoea were noted in 1–1.5%. In the small number of babies with these conditions, the most common predisposition was preterm delivery; a number of other diagnoses were felt to contribute including fetal distress, jaundice, infection, growth retardation and a difficult delivery.

There did not seem to be a specific association between these early symptoms and analgesia. How-

Table 9.3 Percentages of mothers using analgesia who had preterm delivery or a baby of low birth weight (NBT Survey 1990)

Analgesia	<37 weeks		<2.5 kg	
	n	(%)	n	(%)
Pethidine only	29	(4.5)	34	(5.8)
Meptazinol only	4	(5.8)	3	(3.9)
Epidural only	74	(8.4)	79	(9.4)
Diamorphine only	3	(6.5)	3	(5.1)
GA only	95	(25.0)	87	(23.6)

Table 9.4 Percentages of mothers using analgesia with a single agent and neonatal resuscitation (NBT Survey 1990)

	Mothers receiving agent	O$_2$ only	Bag/IPPV[a]	ET[b]
Entonox only	23.0	11.5	4.0	1.0
Pethidine only	6.0	17.7	7.7	1.2
Epidural only	8.5	19.0	6.0	3.0
GA only	3.6	25.5	18.6	19.0

[a]Intermittent positive pressure ventilation.
[b]Endotracheal tube.

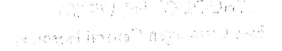

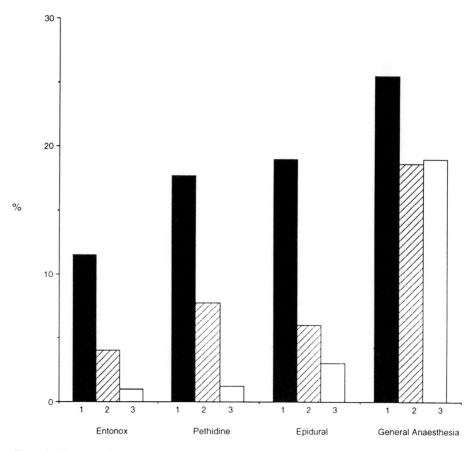

Fig. 9.2   Neonatal resuscitation when mothers used a single analgesic agent (NBT Survey 1990). 1, Oxygen only. 2, Bag/intermittent positive pressure. 3, Endotracheal intubation.

ever, 10.3% of mothers who responded to the question in Branch 2 'Did you think that pain relief affected the baby?' said 'yes' and of these 52.5% said that they thought that the pain relief had made the baby sleepy.

In those babies receiving a single analgesic, pethidine only was associated with the greatest percentage of symptoms noted at the first examination.

> The only thing I did regret was having a pethidine injection which I had only a few minutes before the baby was born. The only effects were that I was drowsy for the next 24 hours and the baby for 48 hours. I was determined to breast feed but could easily have given up as the baby seemed uninterested.

6-WEEK POSTAL FOLLOW-UP

A similar percentage of women (9.5%) as in Branch

2 of the survey thought at 6-week follow-up that the pain relief affected the baby mostly by causing sleepiness; 71% of those women who had reported any problems while another 20% had noticed feeding problems.

At 6 weeks only 2.4% of the babies were reported to be 'mostly difficult' while 71% were 'mostly happy'. 14% of mothers had worries regarding the baby and this was especially noticeable in the mothers who had received a general or epidural anaesthetic.

The reported breast feeding rate was higher than expected, with 50% of babies being breast fed – 42% with breast milk as a sole source of milk. At 6 weeks 43% of the fullterm infants were being breast fed and 29% of the preterm. Similarly, 40.3% of those with normal birth weight and 26.7% of the low birth weight infants were breast fed. The babies of mothers who received Entonox only had a similar breast feeding rate and only a small number were having problems with their babies. Breast feeding rates were less in the group delivered after general anaesthesia and there were more problems.

Among those mothers who were given pethidine, 36% of their babies were being breast fed and 20% had had problems with the baby. The baby's temperament and the mother's confidence with the baby did not seem to be associated with this specific analgesic at 6 weeks, though a greater percentage of mothers were worried about the baby if they had had general or epidural anaesthesia at delivery (24% and 23% respectively). Again the association was likely to have been indirect in that more at-risk babies (including preterm babies) were likely to have been included in these two groups.

The type of analgesia did not have any noticeable effect on the mother's feeling of confidence reported 6 weeks later. However, the more that mothers perceived themselves to be in control at the time of delivery, the more confident they felt with their baby later. 20% of mothers who had pethidine and 14% of those after general anaesthesia thought that there had been side-effects on the baby.

CONCLUSION

The National Birthday Trust survey has demonstrated a number of the expected associations between analgesia and problems in the newborn infant. There was an association between low Apgar scores at 1 and 5 minutes with general anaesthesia although this could at least partly have been due to the fact that more low birth weight babies were delivered by Caesarean section covered by this form of anaesthesia. Pethidine, particularly in combination with other forms of anaesthesia, was associated with decreased Apgar scores at 1 minute and· the same was true of other opiates. Naloxone seemed to be given to a small percentage of all babies, far fewer than the percentage of mothers who received opiate drugs.

The conclusions that one can draw from the findings during the early examination of the baby are clouded by the fact that there were no strict definitions of the conditions reported. Much useful information came from questioning the mother. 10% of those responding although the sample was small in the neonatal period noted an effect of pain relief on the baby, of whom 52% thought that the pain relief had made the baby sleepy. Pethidine was the analgesic associated with the greatest percentage of symptoms noted in a small number at the first examination.

At the 6-week postal follow-up, once again 10% of the women considered that pain relief affected the baby mostly by causing sleepiness and in some cases had caused feeding problems. Breast feeding rates were less in the group delivered after general anaesthesia although 36% of the babies whose mothers had been given pethidine were being breast fed, and 20% of those mothers reporting had problems with the baby.

These findings are reassuring in that the effects of analgesia on the baby were not very striking, and those effects which were found to be associated with general anaesthesia and with epidural anaesthesia might legitimately be attributable to the cause of the instrumental delivery such as low birth weight and low gestation. However, there was noticeably more sleepiness and effect on the baby's feeding behaviour resulting from narcotics. Since narcotic analgesia was one of the most common forms of analgesia used, it would seem that attention needs to be given to this. The dosage, frequency and timing of these agents needs to be carefully controlled. If there is any likelihood of the baby being delivered between 1 and 5 hours after doses of pethidine in excess of 100 mg, then serious consideration should be given to the administration of intramuscular naloxone. Certainly in those babies showing signs of respiratory depression at birth after appropriate resuscitation measures have been employed, naloxone should be given. Perhaps it should also be administered to counteract the late and more prolonged effects of pethidine, sleepiness and interference with feeding (Wiener et al 1977).

Apologies for the delay in replying. My baby has not read the books that say they sleep for X numbers of hours per day and that colic only lasts from 6–10 in the evening!

REFERENCES

Amiel-Tison C, Barrier G, Shnider SM, Levinson G, Hughes S C, Stefani S J 1982 A new neurologic and adaptive capacity scoring system for evaluating obstetric medications in full term infants. Anaesthesiology 56: 340–350

Apgar V, Burns J J, Brodie B B, Papper E M 1952 The transmission of meperidine across the human placenta. American Journal of Obstetrics and Gynecology 64: 1368–1370

Belsey E M et al 1981 The influence of maternal analgesia on neonatal behaviour: I. Pethidine. II. Epidural bupivacaine. British Journal of Obstetrics and Gynaecology 88: 398–413

Brazelton T B 1973 Neonatal behavioural assessment scale. Clinics in Developmental Medicine, 50. Heinemann, London

Broman S, Brackbill Y 1978 Quoted in Kolata G B (author) Behavioural teratology: Birth defects of the mind Science 202: 732–734

Ounsted M 1981 Pain relief during child birth and development at four years. Journal of the Royal Society of Medicine 74: 629–630

Ounsted M, Scott A, Moar V 1980 Delivery and development: to what extent can one associate cause and effect? Journal of the Royal Society of Medicine 73: 786–792

Scanlon J W, Brown W U, Weiss J B, Alper M H 1974 Neurobehavioural responses of newborn infants after maternal epidural anaesthesia. Anaesthesiology 40: 121–128

Wiener P C, Hogg M I, Rosen M 1979 Neonatal respiration, feeding and neurobehavioral state. Effects of intrapartum bupivacaine, pethidine and pethidine reversed by naloxone. Anesthesia 34: 996–1003

Wiener P C, Hogg M I, Rosen M 1977 Effects of naloxone on pethidine induced neonatal depression: I. Intravenous naloxone. II. Intramuscular naloxone. British Medical Journal 2: 228–231

FURTHER READING

Albin M 1987 Fetal and Neonatal effects of analgesia and anaesthetic drugs. In Morgan B (ed) Problems in obstetric anaesthesia. John Wiley, Chichester, pp 177–172

Dailey P A, Baysinger C L, Levinson G, Shnider S M 1982 Neurobehavioural testing of the newborn infant. Clinics in Perinatology 9: 191–214

Hodgkinson R, Marx G F 1981 Effects of analgesia–anaesthesia on the fetus and neonate. In: Cosmi E V (ed) Obstetric anaesthesia and perinatology. Appleton-Century Crofts, pp 451–481

Reynolds F (ed) 1990 Epidural and spinal blockade in obstetrics. Baillière-Tindall, London pp 205–218

10. The follow-up survey

A. Oakley

The topic of pain relief occupies a unique place in the evaluation of the effectiveness of maternity care, for it requires both clinical assessment and a dependence on the subjective feelings of childbearing women. The importance of pain relief within medicine is underlined by the quantity of research on this topic: trials of pharmacological methods of pain relief outnumber all other categories of trials in the perinatal field. In view of this, it is surprising how few studies collect qualitative data. Even fewer attend seriously to methodological and theoretical questions concerning the relationship between pain relief in childbirth and other areas of a woman's experiences to which this may be linked. Most studies which tap women's attitudes are confined to a brief postnatal survey, carried out in hospital and limited to simple questions about satisfaction and to the collection of information about pain experienced, using standardized collection methods. While such an approach may provide valuable data for in-house evaluation of local obstetric analgesic services, it does not allow for women's own evaluations of the relevant and important questions, or permit an assessment of pain relief longitudinally as motherhood proceeds.

Like other important human events, childbirth is an experience which is commonly subject to a good deal of thought and reflection after the event, leading sometimes to substantial re-evaluation of what is considered to have happened. Though such re-evaluations are mediated by the lens of subsequent experience, they could also be taken as an expression of a more considered opinion and interpretation of the sequence of events. It can therefore be argued (as in any attitudinal study) that any comprehensive evaluation of pain in labour and its

relief requires the passage of time to provide essential data. How women feel physically and emotionally in the weeks and months of motherhood after they have left the hospital, and how well and responsive they perceive their babies to be, are part of the information needed by health professionals who are trying to provide a more consumer-sensitive and effective service in the future.

This chapter reports on a postal follow-up to the questions asked of women 6 weeks after birth in the National Birthday Trust survey. A 10% random sample was taken of the original population, and a seven-page questionnaire mailed to these women 6 weeks after delivery. Accompanying the questionnaire was a letter explaining that the purpose of the further questions was to make a comparison between the feelings women have about pain relief immediately after delivery with those some weeks after birth. The letter stressed confidentiality, particularly in relation to any comments the women might wish to express about the hospital or staff who had provided their care.

The questionnaire (see Appendix, Branch 3) contained 26 precoded questions covering the evaluation of pain relief, medical and midwifery care, the general experience of childbirth and motherhood, physical and mental health since, the development and feeding of the baby, the issue of information and choice about pain relief, and plans for a future confinement. The last page of the questionnaire invited women to write additional comments. These are drawn on in the presentation and discussion of data that follow.

Of 1400 questionnaires sent to 10% of all the women in the original survey, 1117 were returned without a reminder. Following one reminder, a further 32 were received. This 82% response rate is in line with other postal surveys of maternity care, recommending this method as a low-cost way of soliciting the opinions of maternity service users. It is also of interest that 46% of the 1149 women returning the follow-up questionnaire responded to the invitation to provide additional comments. An important motivation for completing the questionnaire was referred to by a number of mothers. A typical comment was: 'Thank you for asking me to take part in this survey, if it helps women in the future for better births then that is good'.

The responses to the questionnaire were processed and managed centrally along with the rest of the survey data. For the analysis reported in this chapter, a series of some 500 tabulations was provided, along with texts of the women's comments. The tabulations included some linking from the follow-up questionnaire data (Branch 3) to earlier branches (Branches 1 and 2) of the survey. The tabulations requested were analysed using a Stand Alone statistic pack (using mainly the chi-square test of significance), grouped around the following hypotheses derived from existing work:

1. That women's evaluations of pain experiences would change significantly over time, with the proportion reporting dissatisfaction increasing.
2. That there would be differences between the various methods in terms of their perceived effectiveness at relieving pain, and changes in this assessment over time.
3. That the experience of pain and its relief would be significantly associated with the subsequent physical and emotional experience of motherhood.
4. That pain experiences would be related to aspects of social support and satisfaction with medical and midwifery care, including the extent of information about pain relief.

The discussion which follows is organised around these themes, preceded by a brief presentation of the answers given to the main follow-up questions taken on their own.

SATISFACTION AND OTHER OUTCOMES AT 6 WEEKS

Tables 10.1 and 10.2 give an idea of the pattern of responses at 6 weeks. Table 10.1 relates to general experiences of childbirth and motherhood, and shows that two in three women answering the follow-up questionnaire had enjoyed the birth, though only one in five reported feeling in control either during labour or during delivery.

The questions on control were included in the follow-up questionnaire, as previous work has shown this to be an important dimension of women's experiences of childbearing. It was brought out in many of the unsolicited comments of women completing the Branch 3 follow up questionnaire. Pain relief that maintains a mother's feelings of being in control of what is going on is generally preferable to pain relief that does not facilitate this:

> This is my third child; with my first I had pethidine for pain relief and felt groggy and not *in control*, and after the birth I just wanted to sleep as if I was absolutely exhausted. With my second and third children, I had just gas and air, and I felt completely in control throughout both the labour and the delivery, and afterwards felt great and on a real high, which is how I think it should be.
>
> I had pethidine and gas and air in two previous labours and did not feel I was *in control* at all, so this time I just had gas and air. I felt much more in control and did not notice that the pain was worse.
>
> The epidural I had was given too late – long after I had asked for it – and due to this delay I felt that I lost control whereas at the earlier stages when I was just using breathing I was *in control*.
>
> I didn't feel I needed any pain relief until shortly before the birth. I had chosen meptid and a dose was prepared but my labour progressed much more rapidly than anticipated, so there wasn't time for it to be given. I used Entonox, which seemed to do little more than make me feel dizzy and distant, without aiding the *control* of pain. (I think I had more relief from biting the tube.)

Table 10.1 shows that less than half the women described their physical health as very good in the period since the delivery. The specific incidence of problems reported as a result of the birth (not shown in Table 10.1) was: major discomfort due to stitches 24%; incontinence 22%, dysuria 25%; piles 50%; varicose veins 11%; breast abscess 9%; cracked nipples 35%; and breast engorgement 48%. Some of these problems were recounted in the women's comments, especially as regards the sore topic of perineal sutures:

Table 10.1 Women's experiences of childbirth and motherhood: Follow-up responses (NBT Survey 1990)

Aspect	Response	n	(%)
Enjoyed the birth	Yes	759	(67)
	No	268	(24)
	Don't know/other	101	(9)
Control during labour	Complete	207	(19)
	Some	594	(53)
	Not much/none	286	(26)
	Don't know/other	35	(2)
Control during delivery	Complete	192	(17)
	Some	483	(43)
	Not much/none	420	(38)
	Don't know/other	27	(2)
Physical health since birth	Very well	479	(42)
	Well	540	(48)
	Not very well	112	(10)
	Not at all well	2	(< 1)
Mental health since birth	Very happy	421	(37)
	Happy	577	(51)
	Depressed	89	(8)
	Don't know/other	47	(4)
Confidence as a mother	Very confident	277	(21)
	Quite confident	857	(75)
	Not very/not at all confident	41	(3)
	Don't know/other	3	(< 1)
Baby's temperament	Happy	807	(71)
	Mixed	295	(26)
	Difficult	27	(2)
	Don't know/other	6	(< 1)
Worries about baby	No	968	(85)
	Yes	158	(14)
	Don't know/other	8	(< 1)

The labour and delivery were painful (no pain relief other than breathing exercises and Entonox) but bearable, but the stitches after were absolutely dreadful. I did not have an episiotomy, and a jagged tear resulted from the delivery. The stitches were extremely painful, and it took a long time to insert them. I was given a local anaesthetic (injection) which had no effect whatsoever – and I had to use far more gas and air than I did for the delivery.

Although the pain relief given was great . . . I would say the stitches were worse than the actual labour.

Pain after the birth due to stitches etc. was far worse than the pain during labour and delivery.

The disadvantages of Caesarean section were also cited by many mothers. According to one:

'I unfortunately got an abscess in the centre of the wound which took about 4 weeks to clear, I also had the baby blues, which didn't help much, and I couldn't do the exercises in case the wound opened – because of the abscess it hadn't healed properly afterwards. I am still a bit worried about my bleeding as it still hasn't stopped.

Another woman had other problems in addition to the aftermath of the Caesarean section:

A few days after discharge I had problems with the scar line as I had an abscess . . . It was very painful and took 10 days to heal with help of daily dressings and antibiotics. Throughout the duration of my pregnancy I suffered very severely from hyperemesis gravidarum which led to me losing 3 stone in weight . . . 8 weeks after the birth I still have problems with eating . . . This I find very disappointing and am seeing my GP regularly.

Despite these difficulties, rather more than one in three mothers described their mental health as very good, and one in five said they felt very confident as a mother. Three-quarters described their babies' temperaments as very happy and four out of five reported no particular worries about their babies.

Table 10.2 contains data relating to pain, pain relief and satisfaction. By the time they completed the follow-up survey, one in ten women remembered their labour as pain-free or only slightly painful, one in five remembered having some pain, half severe but bearable pain, and rather less than one in five severe and unbearable pain. By comparison, delivery is recalled as less painful, with one in five women reporting no or very little pain, a third severe but bearable pain and around one in ten severe and unbearable pain. A third of the women described being very satisfied with their pain relief, and only about one in ten dissatisfied or very dissatisfied. Two-thirds said it had been given at the right time, one in five that it had been given too late. The crucial importance of timing was highlighted in many of the women's comments, of which the following are a few:

I was very pleased with the overall birth – midwives were great, very helpful. The epidural was given too late. I found it very hard to keep still on my side in labour with needles being put in my back. Especially when a pain came. It started to take effect after she was born, which was too late and very uncomfortable.

I felt the main thing that made the pain bearable was not the medical pain relief available but the support and encouragement of my husband and midwife plus a sure knowledge of what was happening to my body through antenatal classes. If you know why you feel pain you can cope.

Overall I still feel that giving birth was very painful. My contractions started at every 7 minutes, and they were painful. When I asked for some pain relief, they told me to wait a bit longer. So eventually when I got pain relief (pethidine), I didn't find it much help, and while I was actually giving birth the gas and air made me vomit. Maybe, if they had listened to me when I said the pain was unbearable and gave me pain relief, it might have helped more. But in my case I feel I received it too late.

Pain relief was fine until the last hour after the waters were broken. Then the pain became very severe and I asked for pethidine. I was given half dose of my first pregnancy, which didn't do much good. I was given another dose of the

Table 10.2 Pain, pain relief and satisfaction: follow-up responses (NBT Survey 1990)

Aspect	Response	n	(%)
Pain in labour	Very little/none	110	(10)
	Some	247	(22)
	Bearable severe	552	(49)
	Unbearable severe	178	(16)
	Don't know/other	37	(3)
Pain during delivery	Very little/none	257	(23)
	Some	272	(24)
	Bearable severe	395	(35)
	Unbearable severe	162	(14)
	Don't know/other	41	(4)
Satisfaction with pain relief	Very satisfied	399	(37)
	Satisfied	480	(45)
	Dissatisfied/very dissatisfied	152	(14)
	Don't know	36	(4)
Timing of pain relief	Right time	711	(67)
	Too early	42	(4)
	Too late	204	(19)
	Don't know/other	112	(10)
Satisfaction with midwifery care	Very satisfied	851	(75)
	Satisfied	220	(20)
	Dissatisfied/very dissatisfied	43	(4)
	Don't know	14	(1)
Satisfaction with doctors' care	Very satisfied	435	(39)
	Satisfied	280	(25)
	Dissatisfied/very dissatisfied	65	(6)
	Don't know	48	(4)
	Doctor not present	289	(26)

same amount right at the end which didn't take effect until after my baby was born. Had I been told the delivery was imminent, I wouldn't have asked for the second dose [which] made me feel ill after the birth when I wanted to concentrate on my baby.

This latter comment draws attention to the need for good communication between women and their attendants during labour: decisions about pain relief are intimately linked to stages of labour and delivery, so that what is a good method at one time may not be at another.

As Table 10.2 shows, three-quarters of the women described the care received from midwives as very satisfactory. A smaller proportion, about two in five, said the same about their medical care; fewer women had seen a doctor in labour and, in a quarter of labours, there was no doctor present. There was wide variation in the comments offered in relation to professional care:

The hospital staff were marvellous. We are considering staying in the area for longer than expected so that should we decide to have more children we would be treated by the same people.

I was very pleased and impressed by the care and attention I had from all the staff during my labour and afterwards.

I feel extremely bitter that I was not able to enjoy the birth of my baby, due to neglect on behalf of the midwives. I had only one visit during labour, left in a room on my own. After pleading for pain relief on many occasions I was offered 2 paracetamols. Nobody monitored the progress, so I suffered agony until they realized I was near to delivery, and rushed me to delivery suite. Approximately 20 minutes later, the baby was born. Not a birth I would wish to remember.

During my labour of 16 hours I had care from 5 midwives and 3 doctors. One midwife was unnecessarily threatening, saying things like 'You are not in enough pain', and 'I'm going to really give you some pain'. She then turned my drip from 5 to 40 drops/minute, and insisted on giving me meptid. This treatment caused a lot of stress and upset as I became frightened of her. One doctor stood in the doorway and said 'Give her an epidural, episiotomy and forceps', then walked off. Totally impersonal, and all the things I did not want.

THE EVALUATION OF PAIN EXPERIENCES OVER TIME

It is unfortunately not possible to compare directly mothers' ratings of the painfulness of labour and delivery and satisfaction with pain relief obtained shortly after delivery with those recorded in the follow-up survey, as the same questions were not asked at the two data collection points in Branches 2 and 3. However, Tables 10.3 and 10.4 contain other data for both time periods relating to pain relief and the different methods available, together with a simple quantification of response changes over time. After delivery 70% of women said they felt they had been very free to choose their preferred method of pain relief, a percentage that has fallen to 55% 6 weeks later. Over one-third of women changed the response given to this question after delivery and at 6 weeks. This pattern is similar, though less marked, for adequacy of information: 92% of women after delivery and 82% 6 weeks later say they had enough information about pain relief. Reporting of side-effects on the mother declined from 43% to 20% with nearly half the mothers giving different answers (presumably in part because of the fading of some side-effects with time). The figures are more stable for side-effects noted on the baby (12% after delivery and 10% at 6 weeks).

Of interest in Table 10.3 is not only the comparison of figures across time periods but the absolute levels of satisfaction and dissatisfaction noted; for example, 15% of mothers at 6 weeks said they had not felt at all free to choose the method of pain relief they wanted, and had had inadequate information about pain relief; 20% described the method used as having adversely affected them and 10% their babies. A further 10% reported effects on feeding of the methods of pain relief used (not shown in Table 10.3).

All these dimensions of pain relief are referred to in the women's comments. The mother's right to choose and the importance of full information beforehand are particularly stressed:

I didn't have any choice about pain relief. I was given the pethidine and gas and air. The pethidine made it a little easy, the gas and air made me very wheezy afterwards. I was not consulted on what I would have preferred . . . I thought that everybody had a choice.

When we arrived at the hospital we stated straight away that I wanted an epidural anaesthetic. The nurse tried to jolly us out of it. On the two or three subsequent occasions that I

Table 10.3 Evaluation of pain relief over time: Freedom of choice, information and side effects (NBT Survey 1990)

Aspect	After delivery		At 6 weeks		Same[a]	Neg.[b]	Pos.[c]
	n	(%)	n	(%)	%	%	%
Freedom of choice							
Very free	738	(70)	603	(55)	64	28	9
Quite free	241	(23)	323	(30)			
Not very/not at all free	77	(7)	165	(15)			
Information							
Enough	813	(92)	901	(82)	83	13	4
Not enough	70	(8)	168	(15)			
Don't know	–	–	32	(3)			
Side-effects on woman in hospital							
None	510	(57)	834	(76)	55	12	33
Some	379	(43)	218	(20)			
Don't know/other	–	–	46	(4)			
Side-effects on baby							
None	730	(88)	938	(85)	80	7	12
Some	96	(12)	104	(10)			
Don't know/other	–	–	57	(5)			

[a]Percentage with same response after delivery and at 6 weeks.
[b]Percentage with more negative response at 6 weeks.
[c]Percentage with more positive response at 6 weeks.

> pleaded that the pain was too much to bear I was told to leave it a while and see how it went...I felt my wishes were ignored and that I had no control over what was happening.

A number of women noted that respecting their own decisions could mean a change from choices made before labour:

> I had requested an epidural on my birth plan but at the time my midwife advised me that I was doing well without it (the cervix 5 cm dilated). She left the choice completely up to me and after the birth I was very glad that I had pethidine instead.

Tables 10.4a, b and c disaggregate further this information about pain relief and satisfaction by main methods used, providing comparable data from the two time periods and showing the extent to which women's responses change. As these data are based on any method used, rather than the main or the sole method used, there may be some conflation of effects in the responses. Table 10.4a shows that, for each method, the absolute percentage of women who choose a method for a future delivery at 6 weeks is lower than that reported just after delivery (Branch 2 questionnaire). At 6 weeks the percentages of women choosing the various

methods are 82% relaxation, 76% Entonox, 54% massage, 49% pethidine, 24% TENS and 35% epidural.

So far as side-effects are concerned, the percentages reporting these at 6 weeks are 27% for epidural, 22% relaxation, 19% Entonox and pethidine and 11% TENS for the woman (Table 10.4b). For the baby, the data are 18% pethidine, 13% massage, 11% relaxation, 10% Entonox, 7% TENS and 6% epidural (Table 10.4c). Women who used breathing exercises and relaxation are most likely to give the same response after delivery and 6 weeks later to the question about side-effects on themselves, while users of pethidine and TENS the least likely; for side-effects on the baby the most consistent responders are users of breathing and relaxation, and the least those who had pethidine and Entonox.

PAIN AND THE EXPERIENCE OF MOTHERHOOD

In Table 10.5 the different methods of pain relief are ranked according to the relationship each showed with the main outcomes evaluated in the follow-up questionnaire.

The overall ranking (obtained by adding the

Table 10.4a Evaluation of pain relief over time by different methods. Choice for a future delivery (NBT Survey 1990)

Method	After delivery		At 6 weeks		Same[a] (%)	Neg.[b] (%)	Pos.[c] (%)
	n	(%)	n	(%)			
Breathing exercises/relaxation							
Yes	569	(88)	734	(82)	91	7	2
No	52	(8)	93	(10)			
Don't know	26	(4)	68	(8)			
Massage							
Yes	271	(63)	409	(54)	78	12	10
No	70	(16)	152	(20)			
Don't know	87	(21)	196	(26)			
TENS							
Yes	117	(36)	155	(24)	89	11	0
No	76	(23)	176	(27)			
Don't know	136	(41)	324	(49)			
Entonox							
Yes	677	(83)	743	(76)	94	3	3
No	93	(11)	150	(16)			
Don't know	50	(6)	81	(8)			
Pethidine							
Yes	404	(59)	457	(49)	81	10	9
No	195	(28)	743	(36)			
Don't know	90	(13)	143	(15)			
Epidural							
Yes	286	(47)	314	(35)	89	9	2
No	236	(39)	445	(50)			
Don't know	90	(14)	137	(15)			

[a]Percentage with same response after delivery and at 6 weeks.
[b]Percentage with more negative response at 6 weeks.
[c]Percentage with more positive response at 6 weeks.

individual ranks for each method) is shown across the bottom of Table 10.5. Breathing and relaxation, massage and Entonox are most highly ranked, and pethidine least highly, with TENS and epidural anaesthesia falling inbetween. Of particular interest is the patterning of ranks by the different outcomes for epidural analgesia. This method clearly offers excellent pain relief, but is considerably more negatively evaluated by women in terms of control, side-effects and subsequent physical and emotional health.

As would be expected, these different assessments of pain relief methods are reflected in the women's questionnaire comments. This is particularly the case for pethidine:

> Pethidine at its height was one of the most frightening experiences I have ever had, rendering me unable to communicate with the staff or my husband. I was in a state of semi-awareness, but fully aware of the pain, without the control element of full consciousness. Had I not had the pethidine, I would have been able to explain to the midwife that I was already in the second stage of labour when the epidural was given.
>
> I now feel that I failed in some way because I had pethidine so close to the delivery of my baby. I had only wanted to use gas and air but felt I couldn't cope on it alone at the time, but felt that had I received more encouragement (verbal) from the midwives in attendance I could have managed on gas and air alone. I didn't feel all that confident in their handling of me, and had I done so I'd have managed without pethidine, I'm sure. I've been left with this feeling that I'd like to do it again because I'm sure I'd do it differently and better. I didn't like the effect the pethidine had on my baby, which resulted in her being taken away from me almost immediately, and I felt responsible. I think in a nutshell what I mean is that the psychological care of the mother is the most important aspect of pain management in most cases. Had I not had pethidine I would have felt better both about myself and the baby.

In some cases, the comments on pethidine refer to a previous birth:

Table 10.4b Evaluation of pain relief over time by different method — perceived side-effects on the mother (NBT Survey 1990)

Method	After delivery		At 6 weeks		Same[a]	Neg.[b]	Pos.[c]
	n	(%)	n	(%)	(%)	(%)	(%)
Breathing exercises/relaxation							
No	34	(63)	320	(74)	67	11	22
Yes	16	(30)	96	(22)			
Don't know	4	(7)	17	(4)			
Massage							
No	55	(63)	168	(79)	66	11	23
Yes	29	(33)	42	(20)			
Don't know	3	(4)	4	(1)			
TENS							
No	33	(54)	58	(83)	51	11	38
Yes	27	(44)	16	(21)			
Don't know	1	(2)	1	(2)			
Entonox							
No	313	(64)	540	(79)	58	8	34
Yes	158	(32)	127	(19)			
Don't know	20	(4)	19	(2)			
Pethidine							
No	158	(46)	331	(78)	56	7	37
Yes	173	(50)	80	(19)			
Don't know	15	(4)	13	(3)			
Epidural							
No	62	(58)	140	(70)	59	17	24
Yes	41	(39)	57	(27)			
Don't know	3	(3)	4	(3)			

[a]Percentage with same response after delivery and at 6 weeks.
[b]Percentage with more negative response at 6 weeks.
[c]Percentage with more positive response at 6 weeks.

> Both I and my husband have said this birth was much better to handle and be more in control of than my other child's birth where I had pethidine. Though at the time I was in a great deal of pain, I felt the pethidine sent me to sleep for most of my labour, and I found great difficulty in the actual birth, and ended up with forceps. I started off quite depressed and found great difficulty in coping with my child for quite some time, physically and emotionally.

Pain and attitudes to pain relief are shown in Table 10.6 by some of the main aspects of women's experiences of motherhood and by satisfaction with medical and midwifery care. Most of the variables included in this table are interrelated, as shown in the high proportion (85%) of statistically significant chi-square results. Of the variables relating to motherhood on the left-hand side of Table 10.6, maternal confidence and perception of the baby's temperament are least likely to be significantly associated with pain and its relief. Conversely, and as would be expected, enjoyment of labour and feelings of control appear to be intimately linked. The impact on physical health seems to be stronger than that on emotional health.

SOCIAL SUPPORT

The value of continuity of care and the support of midwives were especially singled out in the women's comments:

> A friendly nurse holding your hand goes a long way to helping with pain and giving you reassurance. The nurses made you feel great, giving you individual attention and time to talk about any pain you may be in.
>
> The labour was very long and painful, but under the Domino scheme I saw the same midwife most of the time and found this an enormous help in labour as this gave me confidence.

Social support was also noted for its absence, along with other developments in modern maternity care:

Table 10.4c Evaluation of pain relief over time by different methods. Perceived side-effects on baby (NBT Survey 1990)

Method	After delivery		At 6 weeks		Same[a]	Neg.[b]	Pos.[c]
	n	(%)	n	(%)	(%)	(%)	(%)
Breathing exercises/relaxation							
No	43	(80)	368	(85)	94	2	4
Yes	6	(11)	49	(11)			
Don't know	5	(9)	18	(4)			
Massage							
No	68	(77)	171	(80)	91	3	6
Yes	11	(13)	28	(13)			
Don't know	9	(10)	15	(7)			
TENS							
No	51	(81)	63	(89)	92	3	5
Yes	5	(8)	5	(7)			
Don't know	7	(11)	3	(4)			
Entonox							
No	466	(79)	582	(85)	89	5	6
Yes	62	(11)	69	(10)			
Don't know	65	(10)	35	(5)			
Pethidine							
No	237	(68)	315	(74)	85	7	8
Yes	61	(18)	78	(18)			
Don't know	51	(14)	31	(8)			
Epidural							
No	91	(85)	182	(90)	95	2	3
Yes	6	(6)	13	(6)			
Don't know	10	(9)	7	(4)			

[a]Percentage with same response after delivery and at 6 weeks.
[b]Percentage with more negative response at 6 weeks.
[c]Percentage with more positive response at 6 weeks.

Table 10.5 Ranking of different methods of pain relief by maternally reported outcomes (NBT Survey 1990)

	Breathing/relaxation (n = 449)	Massage (n = 220)	TENS (n = 71)	Entonox (n = 689)	Pethidine (n = 424)	Epidural (n = 202)	p value
Enjoyment of labour	2	1	6	3	4	5	$p<0.05$
Control in labour	2	1	5	3	4	6	$p<0.0001$
Control during delivery	2	1	5	3	4	6	$p<0.0001$
Pain in labour	2	4	6	3	5	1	$p<0.0001$
Pain during delivery	3	2	4	5	6	1	$p<0.0001$
Satisfaction with pain relief	2	3	6	4	5	1	$p<0.001$
Side-effects: women in hospital	5	4	1	2	3	6	NS
women at home	4	3	5	1	2	6	$p<0.0001$
Side-effects: baby	3	5	4	2	6	1	$p<0.0001$
feeding	3	2	5	4	6	1	$p=0.05$
Physical health	1	2	3	4	5	6	$p=0.05$
Mental health	3	2	1	4	5	6	$p<0.0001$
Confidence as a mother	5	3	6	1	4	2	NS
Baby's temperament	2	1	4	5	6	3	NS
Worries about baby	1	2	6	3	4	5	NS
Choice for future delivery	1	4	6	2	5	3	$p<0.0001$
Overall ranking	2	1	5	3	6	4	

Table 10.6 Pain, pain relief and satisfaction by maternal outcomes and obstetric/midwifery care factors (NBT Survey 1990)

	Satisfaction with pain relief	Timing of pain relief	Freedom of choice	Pain in labour	Pain in delivery
Enjoyment of labour	$p < 0.0001$	$p < 0.0001$	$p < 0.0001$	$p < 0.0001$	$p < 0.0001$
Control in labour	$p < 0.0001$	$p < 0.0001$	$p < 0.0001$	$p < 0.0001$	$p < 0.0001$
Control in delivery	$p < 0.0001$	$p < 0.0001$	$p < 0.0001$	$p < 0.0001$	$p < 0.0001$
Confidence as mother	$p < 0.001$	NS	$p < 0.005$	NS	$p < 0.0001$
Emotional health	$p < 0.0001$	$p < 0.001$	$p < 0.001$	$p = 0.01$	NS
Worries about baby	$p < 0.05$	$p < 0.05$	NS	$p < 0.0001$	$p < 0.0001$
Baby's temperament	$p = 0.05$	NS	NS	$p < 0.05$	NS
Mother's physical health	$p < 0.0001$	$p < 0.005$	$p < 0.0005$	$p < 0.0001$	$p < 0.0001$
Satisfaction with midwives' care	$p < 0.0001$	$p < 0.0001$	$p < 0.005$	$p < 0.005$	$p < 0.05$
Satisfaction with doctors' care	$p < 0.0001$	$p < 0.0001$	$p < 0.0001$	$p < 0.005$	$p < 0.0001$
Continuity of care	$p < 0.0001$	NS	NS	$p < 0.0001$	$p < 0.0001$
Choice of place of delivery for next baby	$p < 0.0001$	$p < 0.0001$	$p < 0.0001$	$p < 0.01$	$p < 0.01$

I think that what I would have liked most in labour was someone just to talk to . . . The first time . . . 4 years ago was great, lots of midwives and nurses to talk to, which helped me take my mind off things. This time the poor midwives were so busy. There is not enough staff. I would have liked to have stayed in hospital longer, but they had to move three of us into a closed ward on the second day as they needed our beds downstairs. We were made to feel we had to go home. It was not as happy a stay as I had 4 years ago.

Not surprisingly, continuity of care proved to be significantly associated ($p < 0.05$, not tabulated) with the desire to be delivered in the same place next time.

The direction of the association for most of the variables shown in Table 10.6 is as expected, i.e. high satisfaction, satisfaction with timing, and perception of free choice are associated with high levels of enjoyment, control, confidence, with medical and midwifery care satisfaction, and with fewer worries about the baby and perception of her or him as anything other than happy. Pain in labour and delivery does, however, show a more complex relationship with these aspects of motherhood; the highest proportions of women reporting positive experiences are to be found in the groups experiencing some or very little pain, and not in the category reporting none. The incidence of positive experiences among women recalling a great deal of bearable pain is also relatively high – for example, 71% of those whose delivery pain fell in this category said they enjoyed the birth.

The social context of childbirth as reflected in occupational and marital status, partner support and antenatal education is shown in Table 10.7. It is of interest that although social class is unrelated to satisfaction with pain relief, it is related to perceptions of freedom of choice and adequacy of information (with more working class women feeling unfree and inadequately informed). Antenatal education appears to increase the chances of a woman feeling free to choose.

Table. 10.7 Social class, support and pain relief satisfaction (NBT Survey 1990)

	Satisfaction with pain relief	Timing of pain relief	Freedom of choice	Information
Social class:				
woman	NS	$p < 0.0001$	NS	$p < 0.0001$
man	NS	NS	$p < 0.0001$	NS
Marital status	NS	NS	NS	NS
Support of partner	NS	$p < 0.0005$	NS	$p < 0.05$
Antenatal education	NS	$p < 0.05$	$p < 0.05$	NS

Associations with obstetric and paediatric factors are shown in Table 10.8. Whereas the delivery method, the onset of labour and the baby's admission to the neonatal unit are not significantly associated with pain relief satisfaction, whether a woman had a spontaneous onset of labour is associated with her perception of control during labour. Delivery method is associated with the enjoyment of birth, feelings of control, and the woman's emotional health and worries about the baby 6 weeks later. Predictably, the baby's admission to the neonatal unit is also linked with an increase in negative experiences for the mother, either because both are associated with some common determining factor, or because what happens to the baby after birth colours remembrance of earlier events. In the women's comments on the questionnaires, these connections were mentioned, particularly with respect to Caesarean birth:

> I did not think there was enough information given at the hospital and antenatal classes about Caesarean birth. I found out at 37 weeks that my baby was a breech. I was very shocked when they told me it would be a Caesarean birth. I was very frightened, I tried to read up on it but there wasn't much information about it, they told you about before the operation, but not what to expect afterwards. For example, the pain from the stitches and not being able to move because of the pain. So you can't do things for yourself, and your bowels don't work properly and that you cannot have a proper meal for 48 hours after. On the second day in hospital I remember crying because I couldn't get over the shock of what had happened. I just felt like I had missed out. I'd had

> one good birth with my first child, and it was brilliant, no stitches or complications, so I know I should be thankful, but I can't. Last time I could do exercises because the hospital gave me an exercise sheet, this time when I asked for some information on exercises I got told that I had to take it easy, so I still don't know what exercises I can do. To me it feels like nobody is bothered about a section birth or how the mother feels before and after. I mean even in your survey there's only one question about it.

CONCLUSION

It has only been possible to discuss some of the data which were related to social and medical factors obtained in the follow-up survey on women's perceptions of pain and its relief. More sophisticated and extensive analyses will eventually be produced, involving more data linkages between the various branches of the survey as a whole. The limitations of the present analysis should be borne in mind, particularly as regards the likelihood that using chi-squared tests of significance in a large number of tables will generate some spurious significant associations. Conversely, a non-significant association may well be meaningful in real life, as in the example of partner support, which, although a feature of labour many women consider important, proved to be statistically unrelated either to satisfaction with pain relief or to other outcomes.

Despite these caveats, the data presented here do justify some important conclusions. Most women

Table 10.8 Evaluation of birth experience at 6 weeks by obstetric variables (NBT Survey 1990)

	Percentages of women reporting				
	Enjoyment of birth	Control in labour	Control in delivery	Emotional health	Worries
Onset of labour					
Spontaneous	71	22	19	41	13
Induced	63	15	15	32	15
	NS	$p < 0.0001$	NS	$p = 0.06$	NS
Delivery method					
Spontaneous	73	22	21	39	13
Assisted	56	7	2	43	14
LSCS	40	3	3	31	26
	$p < 0.0001$	$p < 0.0001$	$p < 0.0001$	$p < 0.05$	$p < 0.0001$
Baby's admission to NNU					
No	69	19	18	42	14
Yes	52	8	6	39	21
	$p = 0.05$	$p < 0.0001$	$p < 0.0001$	$p < 0.001$	NS

say they are satisfied with the care relating to the relief of pain in labour, a finding which is in line with other research on consumer satisfaction. In this respect, maternity patients are no different from other health care users of the same sex and age. In any measurement of satisfaction, there is an inbuilt bias towards the status quo; that is, questions about satisfaction are not likely to tap people's visions of more radical alternatives.

Despite the usual bias towards satisfaction exhibited in these responses, it is important to note that a significant proportion of women are not content with the state of affairs regarding pain relief experienced during their labours and deliveries; 14% were dissatisfied with their pain relief, and 23% said it had been given at the wrong time; 15% had not felt free to choose, and the same percentage had not been given adequate information. More than a third of the women said they did not feel in control of their deliveries, and one in four said this of labour. One in ten mothers experienced impaired physical and mental health in the early weeks of motherhood, some of which was clearly identified by them as consequent on use of a particular method or methods of pain relief. The incidence of physical health problems was considerable, with one in five women reporting incontinence, perineal discomfort due to stitches, and dysuria, half piles, one in three cracked nipples, and a half reporting breast engorgement. Breakdown of women's responses by the different pain relief methods used supports other work showing pethidine to be a particularly problematic method of pain relief, and also supports research suggesting that although epidural analgesia offers good pain relief it also has deleterious psychological and physical effects on women's health.

The social context in which women have babies is important in particular ways. Although social class is unrelated to satisfaction with pain relief, the association with freedom of choice and information shown in Table 10.7 replicates Cartwright's finding that working-class women have more unasked questions about childbirth and maternity care than middle-class women. A striking feature of the women's comments overall is that their evaluations of pain relief typically combine a mixture of different considerations – not only the efficacy of the method in relieving pain at the time, but its impact on their feelings about their own role in their birth then and in the months afterwards, possible effects on maternal and infant health, and on feeding. It is difficult to reflect the holistic approach evident in women's approaches to pain in childbirth in simple questions about satisfaction. Indeed, this is a problem that has bedevilled the interpretation and measurement of pain and its meanings for many years; traditional approaches suffer from a division between the physical and the emotional which is not reflected in people's experiences.

A critical aspect of experiences relating to pain and its relief for childbearing women is the relation between past and present events for those who have had children before; central to this is the changing expectations many women may find they learn to have. As one mother put it:

> This is my second child and as such I feel more confident about her management and knew what to expect in labour. I didn't need much help or advice as I had already learned by my mistakes this time. My expectations of help were greater with my first child but not fulfilled.

Another said:

> As this is my third baby I felt confident about most aspects of motherhood. I had a planned section with this baby; the other two were normal deliveries. If I had filled in this form after having my first baby, it would have been completely different. I didn't feel there was much help or information available to first time mothers. You were just left to learn through experience as I have done.

When different births take place in very different circumstances, the nature of the comparison that can be made may be quite fundamental:

> My baby was born at home 6 weeks ago. My first child was born in hospital 2 years ago. The difference between the two births is immense, also the care given. In hospital the confidence of the parents is undermined; I'm convinced there is a tendency to interfere in the natural birth process – giving control to the staff for example, rupturing membranes, timing events, excessive monitoring, speeding up labour . . . if one thing happens such as an epidural . . . other things have to happen such as forceps delivery. My last

labour was 24 hours – most at hospital. I found it a long and tiring experience but still enjoyed it. However, I found the staff irritating, contradicting each other's advice, undermining my confidence . . . At home I felt in control, didn't need any pain relief . . . We were all relaxed and happy, the care given was brilliant. Hospitals seem to dramatise a very natural experience. However, in an emergency they are definitely needed and work well. I felt I got much more care at home.

One mother was critical of the orientation of the questionnaire itself, expressing the view that it was:

. . . very much geared towards hospital birth and medical forms of pain relief, i.e. pethidine, epidural, gas and air. I had a home birth with the independent midwives, without the above forms of pain relief, because I believe pain is part of childbirth. The forms of pain relief I used were being able to move around, yelling, massage, a bath, and being at home in my own environment where I felt relaxed and calm.

This is despite the fact that the form also asked questions about non-pharmacological methods such as massage, relaxation exercises and TENS.

Although many of the comments were positive and constructive, some women used the questionnaire to tell very sad stories, indicative of low levels of support and help. All such accounts are, as the Short Committee put it a number of years ago, evidence of failure on the part of the maternity services to provide women with a good experience at the same time as pursuing the goal of a healthy baby:

. . . what I would like to know is why my children have all been early, and why is it when you go for a scan round about 7 months and no-one can tell you what you are having? I think it's a woman's right, after all, that's why a lot of mothers who are pregnant with their second and third babies don't come for antenatal. We should be given the choice, and in my opinion the best pain relief any one can have is having someone you love very much at your side, and if you have a premature baby you should be able to stay in with the baby no matter how many children there are at home, because coming home without that baby hurts more than anything in this world. We might put on a smile going home, but once we leave hospital you feel as if you've lost that baby. Please think about us, we are the mothers . . .

REFERENCES

Bendelow G 1992 Perceptions of pain and gender. PhD thesis, University of London
Cartwright A 1964 Human relations and hospital care. Routledge and Kegan Paul, London
Cartwright A 1979 The dignity of labour? Tavistock, London
Cartwright A 1987 Monitoring maternity services by postal questionnaires to mothers. Health Trends 19: 19–20
Dickersin K 1989 Pharmacological control of pain during labour. In: Chalmers I, Enkin M, Keirse M J N C (eds) Effective care in pregnancy and childbirth. Oxford University Press, Oxford
Garel M, Crost M 1982 L'analgesie peridurale: le point de vue des femmes. Gynecol. Obstet. Biol. Reprod. Vol 11: 523–533
Green J, Coupland V, Kitzinger J 1988 Great expectations; a prospective study of women's expectations and experiences of childbirth. Unpublished report, Child Care and Development Group, Cambridge
Murray A D, Dolby R M, Nation R F, Thomas D B 1981 Effects of epidural anaesthesia on newborns and their mothers. Child Development 52: 71–82
National Perinatal Epidemiology Unit 1986 A classified bibliography of controlled trials in perinatal medicine 1940–1984. Oxford University Press, Oxford.
Oakley A 1980 Women confined: towards a sociology of childbirth. Martin Robertson, Oxford
Oakley A, Rajan L, Grant A 1990 Social support and pregnancy outcome; report of a randomized trial. British Journal of Obstetrics and Gynaecology 97: 155–162
Porter M, Macintyre S 1984 What is must be best. Social Science and Medicine 19: 1197–1200
Riley E D M 1977 What do women want? The question of choice in the conduct of labour. In: Chard T, Richards M P M (eds) Benefits and hazards of the new obstetrics. Spastics international medical publications, London
Short Committee 1980 (Second report from the Social Services Committee) Perinatal and neonatal mortality. HMSO, London
Williams S, Hepburn M, McIlwaine G 1985 Consumer view of epidural analgesia. Midwifery 1: 32–36

11. Findings and recommendations of the NBT Survey

G. Chamberlain,   A. Wraight,   P. Steer

These are the recommendations of the organisers of the survey and editors of the report. They do not represent the views of the National Birthday Trust of necessity, but since the editors had spent much time considering the data, their opinions may be helpful.

FINDINGS

ORGANISATIONAL

1. The National Birthday Trust has performed five national surveys since the Second World War; over 95% of the information was provided by midwives. On this occasion, only 88% of delivery units were able to join and the midwives who covered virtually every delivery in the country only reported data on 66% of the women delivered.

2. Women who have had stillbirths or sick babies do want to be included in surveys.

3. Government statistics about maternity matters are incomplete for some years in the 1980s.

OBSTETRIC FINDINGS

1. 99.5% of women in the survey delivered in hospital.

2. The number of isolated GP delivery units in the UK continues to fall – from 199 in 1984 to 58 in 1990.

3. 20% of women still deliver in obstetric units without consultant obstetric cover.

4. The major obstetric interventional changes noted since the 1984 NBT survey were a fall in the induction rate and a rise in the Caesarean section rate.

ANALGESIA

Background

1. A wide variety of pain-relieving methods are available and used in the UK.

2. Most women use some form of pain relief in labour.

3. Midwives are the major professional group advising women about analgesia in labour.

4. The major determinants of the use of pain relief are the method planned by the woman and the duration of labour. These are modulated by the mode of onset of labour (women are more likely to use analgesia if labour is induced) and the parity of the woman – women in their second or susbequent labour require less analgesia, probably because of greater confidence and a shorter labour.

5. The method of analgesia planned had no significant correlation with the mode of delivery. However, mode of delivery had a highly significant correlation with the method of analgesia used. The spontaneous delivery rate in women using epidurals was only 55% compared with 85% of women using other methods. Both the mode of delivery and use of epidural anaesthesia are strongly related to the duration of labour, and so the relationship is not necessarily cause and effect.

6. Teenagers are more likely to be unsupported and anxious but less likely to have a Caesarean section than the rest of the population.

7. Women over 35 years are increasingly likely to have both medical problems and require a Caesarean section than younger women.

Entonox

Entonox is the most widely available and used

method of pain relief; it is available in 99% of maternity units and used by 60% of women.

Pethidine

1. Pethidine is available in 98% of maternity units and is used by 37% of women.

2. Pethidine has side-effects on mother and baby which make it less than ideal for many women; in particular it can cause confusion and loss of control in the mother and sleepiness in the baby after birth. It is associated with a reduction in the proportion of babies who successfully establish breast feeding.

3. The analgesic effect of pethidine was overrated by midwives.

Diamorphine

This addictive drug is still being used, mostly in Scotland. Its continued use in hospitals puts it at risk for theft for heroin has an active criminal market.

Epidural

1. Epidural analgesia is only available in 63.3% of maternity units, i.e. it is not available in 36.7%.

2. About 18% of women overall use epidural anaesthesia in labour while in units where it is fully available, it is used by 25%.

3. Couples should be told in the antenatal period of the non-availability of epidurals in certain centres. In others they must be told it is available only for certain limited time periods when anaesthetists are present in the hospital.

4. The use of epidural anaesthesia exceeds 50% in women labouring longer than 16 hours with their first baby.

5. Almost half of all women having a Caesarean section had the operation performed under epidural anaesthesia.

6. Epidural anaesthesia is a most effective method of pain relief, but it has more significant side-effects than non-pharmacological methods.

7. The condition of the baby, as measured by the Apgar score, was much better when epidural anaesthesia was used for operative delivery than when other methods were used, especially general anaesthesia.

8. Women were particularly anxious in labour if they had been expecting an epidural but then could not have one.

9. With the reduction of anaesthetic training posts at registrar and senior registrar level, more delivery units will be deprived of this method of analgesia. Women should know this.

Non-pharmacological methods

1. A small percentage of women used alternative methods.

2. Only a very small number of women use TENS; it is probably not very effective and a higher proportion or women using it rated it negatively than those using any other method.

3. TENS equipment was not available or was not working in many units.

Perineal repair

Pain associated with perineal repair after tears or an episiotomy is often severe and many women feel that the analgesic methods available for this procedure are inadequate.

ASSESSMENT OF PAIN

1. The majority of mothers were very happy with the analgesia they used.

2. Poor communication was the most usual reason for dissatisfaction.

3. If not happy, the main reason was that an epidural had been promised but not given.

4. Approximately 50% of women achieved their chosen method of analgesia; if not, there was a feeling of failure and loss of control.

5. Nulliparae tended to use more analgesia than planned, and multiparae less. This was probably a function of the duration of labour.

6. 93.5% of women say they had severe or unbearable pain in labour, when asked shortly after delivery. However, when asked 6 weeks later, this proportion had fallen to 65%.

INFORMATION ABOUT PAIN RELIEF

1. Information about pain relief is obtained from a wide variety of sources, and the source has very little influence on the method chosen.

2. Most women say they are satisfied with the pain relief they received in labour.

GENERAL

1. Feeling in control during labour is an important part of having a positive recollection of childbirth.

2. Pain relief was sometimes given too late because the stage of labour was underestimated.

3. If there are no problems with mother or baby, then the majority of pain relief methods will not cause adverse effect.

4. Pethidine may result in drowsiness of the baby causing difficulties in feeding and interactions with parents.

RECOMMENDATIONS

INFORMATION COLLECTION

1. Government should pay more heed to its statistical services encouraging RHAs to fund and then demand a full data collection service from all DHAs and Trusts.

2. Obstetric units should each have better data collection methods; 56 of 293 units surveyed could not tell us, in the March of one year, what the perinatal mortality rate was in the previous year. We hope these will improve with the audit promised by the new Health Sevice (nHS).

3. Many midwives are disillusioned about data collection because, with the regrading and then the reorganisation of the nHS, they are grossly overworked. Further surveys should involve designated senior midwives only with help to fill in questionnaires.

4. Recently delivered women are not keen to complete even a short questionnaire after leaving hospital, although stamped addressed envelopes are provided. They do have things to do in these busy days other than fill in questionnaires. The 66% response that the National Birthday Trust obtained shows this. When the subset of the same women were re-assayed 6 weeks later, an 82% response was obtained. We recommend that non-supervised questionnaires are not sent to women in the immediate time after delivery.

5. Obstetric services should be centralised and we should continue to close small units unless they are geographically necessary. Staffing, skills and equipment are not available to cover all sites to provide a level of service and safety requested by many mothers; this is exemplified by the epidural anaesthesia service.

EDUCATION

1. The nature and severity of pain in labour should be explained to all pregnant women in a manner understandable to each individually. Full information about all the methods of pain relief available at the place of planned delivery should be discussed with potential mothers and their partners.

2. More effort should be made to provide this information as part of antenatal preparation, irrespective of whether women choose to attend antenatal classes.

3. Every effort must be made to ensure that if methods such as epidural anaesthesia are discussed and accepted, they are available for a full 24-hour service. Even more women should be encouraged to use epidural anaesthesia for operative deliveries, particularly Caesarean sections.

4. Continuing surveillance of women's satisfaction with analgesia methods available at every place of delivery should be undertaken. Managers must allow sufficient funding for this to be part of the normal unit routine.

SPECIFIC MEASURES

1. Research is needed into ways of reducing the side-effects of pethidine, particularly in relation to breast feeding.

2. Improved methods of pain relief for perineal repair are needed.

3. Non-medical volunteers, themselves having had babies, should be available to be with women throughout labour to provide emotional support, particularly to the very young or the unsupported.

4. There is an urgent need for a National Ethics Committee to advise on nationwide research.

FURTHER WORK

1. Another national survey on pain relief in labour should be prepared in 10 years' time to check changes.

Glossary

accoucheur A man acting as a midwife (historic)

acidosis A condition characterised by an accumulation of acids in the blood

acupuncture Stimulation of channels by the insertion of needles into the skin at specific points of the body to treat disorders of organs and alleviate pain

alkalosis An abnormal increase of alkali in the blood

amniotic membranes The inner layer of the fetal sac

anaesthetist Doctor who specialises in the administration of anaesthetics

analgesic A drug that relieves pain

antepartum haemorrhage Bleeding from the genital tract any time between the 28th week of pregnancy and the birth of the baby. From October 1992 this has become 24 weeks

Apgar score A weighted scoring system devised to assess the condition of the baby at birth

aorta The main vessel in the arterial network which carries oxygenated blood from the heart

apnoea Absence of breathing

aromatherapy Use of massage and fragrant oils to relieve the pain of labour

artificial rupture of the membranes Deliberate breaking of the amniotic sac to induce or start labour or to augment it once started naturally

associate specialist Senior doctor with similar training background to a consultant but without full clinical responsibility

augmentation Acceleration of labour following a spontaneous onset to increase the efficiency of uterine contractions when progress is slow

bag and mask resuscitation Manual revival of the baby using a refillable bag and close fitting face mask to force air or oxygen into the lungs

barbiturate Drug used as sedative or hypnotic

brainstorming Intensive discussion to generate ideas or solve problems

breast engorgement Painful accumulation of secretions in the breast often accompanied by venous and lymphatic stasis

breech Delivery in which baby's buttocks present first

brow A head presentation of the fetus at delivery in which the attitude of the head is midway between flexion and extension. It usually requires a Caesarean section for delivery

bupivacaine (Marcain) Long-lasting local anaesthetic often prescribed for epidural block

caesarean section Operation by which the baby is delivered through an incision in the abdominal and uterine walls

cardiac Pertaining to the heart

cervix Neck of the uterus or womb

chi-squared test Test used to compare observed and expected frequencies. The number of cases in the sample needs to be large

chloroform An inhalation used to produce general anaesthesia

clinical assistant A part or full-time post held by less experienced doctors supervised by senior hospital staff. Many such posts are held by GPs wishing to keep up some special aspects of their hospital learnt skills

coccyx Small triangular bone at the base of the vertebral column

compound A presentation of more than one part of the baby in labour, e.g. head and hand

consultant Specialist doctor in an NHS hospital who is ultimately responsible for the management of women admitted to hospital under his care. He directs the policies of the medical teams

correlation coefficient The measure of the closeness of a relationship

cross tabulation Comparison of frequency results of one factor with another

delivery The birth of the baby

diabetes Disease caused by deficient secretion of insulin

diamorphine Strong, long-lasting analgesic given to relieve the pain of labour

dysmenorrhoea Difficult or painful menstruation

endorphins Substances naturally produced in the body in response to acute pain

endotracheal tube A tube passed into the baby's trachea to enable artificial expansion of the lungs

Entonox A 50% mix of nitrous oxide and oxygen, premixed in a cylinder and used as inhalational analgesic

epidural A local anaesthetic injected around the spinal sac causing temporary numbness and loss of sensation in the lower part of the body. It is used in labour to abolish the pain of uterine contractions, or as an alternative to general anaesthetic during Caesarean section

ether A compound used as a general anaesthetic

face presentation Cephalic presentation in which the spine and head of the baby are extended so that the face lies lowest in the pelvis and delivers first

fetus Term given to the baby from 8 weeks of gestation until birth

forceps delivery Method of assisting the delivery of the baby in the second stage of labour by application of suitably curved metal spoon-like blades to the sides of the baby's head

frequency table Simple counts of the number of respondents to have given a particular answer to a question. This needs to be done for every question

general anaesthetic Agents given to a patient to bring about complete loss of consciousness and consequent unawareness of any painful stimuli

general practitioner A family doctor with total overall care of his patients. He is a primary health practitioner but may have extra experience and qualifications in different specialties, e.g. obstetrics

gestation Pregnancy

gravidity Refers to the number of pregnancies a woman has had irrespective of their outcome, i.e. all babies live or stillborn plus miscarriages, induced terminations of pregnancy and ectopic pregnancies

health centre A medical centre placed strategically in the community to provide the full range of primary health care including antenatal care and education

homeopathy Herbal medicine used in very small doses to relieve the pain of labour

hypertension Abnormally high blood pressure

hypnosis A state of apparent deep sleep in which a person acts only under the influence of some external suggestion

hypocapnia An abnormally low arterial carbon dioxide level

hypodermic Subcutaneous

hypoglycaemia Abnormally low blood sugar

hypothermia A fall in the body temperature to subnormal level

hypotonia Deficient muscle tone

hypoxia Lack of oxygen delivered to the body tissues

induction Procedure to artificially start labour where prolongation of the pregnancy would put the health of mother or fetus at risk

intermittent positive pressure ventilation (IPPV) A method of mechanical ventilation to prevent prolonged apnoea

intervillus space Space between the chorionic villi beneath the placenta. Acts as a reservoir for oxygenated maternal blood

intrapartum During labour

intrauterine growth retardation Delay in fetal growth resulting in the baby being small for gestational age

intubation Insertion of a breathing tube through the mouth or nose to ensure a patent airway

in utero transfer Transfer of the mother, before delivery of the baby, to another place of confinement where specialised care can be given to her and her baby before and after birth

labour The delivery process, which takes place in three stages: first–opening of the neck of the uterus (cervix); second – birth of the baby; third – expulsion of the afterbirth

lidocaine A local anaesthetic agent

lignocaine Drug used for local analgesia and nerve block

low birth weight A weight of 2.5 kg or less at birth

massage Rubbing and kneading of back muscles to relieve the pain of labour

mean The average value

median Occupying a position midway between two extremes of a set of values of data

menopause Period during which a woman's menstrual cycle ends.

meptazinol (Meptid) Short-term drug used to relieve the pain of labour.

methoxyflurane (Penthrane) Method of inhalational analgesia for the relief of pain in labour, popular in the 1970s

midazolam (Hypnovel) A parenteral central nervous depressant prescribed for preoperative sedation

midwife One who specialises in the care of women during pregnancy, childbirth and the puerperium

minute volume The total ventilation per minute measured by expired gas collection for a period of 1–3 minutes

mode A value in a set of data that occurs more frequently than other values

monitor A machine which records and displays continuously the rate of the fetal heart.

morphine Strong, long-lasting analgesic

multipara A woman who has given birth to a baby (live or stillborn)

multivariate analysis Method used to correlate one variable with several others

naloxone (Narcan) Drug given to baby to counteract respiratory depression caused by the mother having pethidine or other respiratory depressant in labour

National Childbirth Trust A charity which runs a network of antenatal classes, breast–feeding counselling and postnatal support

neonatal death Death of a baby within 28 days of birth. If such a death occurs in the first 7 days, it is categorised as an early neonatal death; such early deaths are grouped with stillbirths to derive the perinatal mortality rate

neonatal unit A special ward or intensive care nursery which provides continuous skilled supervision of sick newborn babies

neurological Pertaining to the nervous system

nitrous oxide A non-toxic inhalation analgesic used in conjunction with oxygen in labour

nullipara A woman who has never given birth to a baby

obstetrician A doctor who specialises in the care of pregnant women in pregnancy, at their deliveries and in the postnatal period

occipito anterior Presentation when the back of the baby's head is to the front of the mother's pelvis as the head descends through the birth canal

occipito posterior Presentation when the back of the baby's head is towards the back of the mother's pelvis

opiate/opioid Any narcotic or sedative drug

ovary One of the pair of female gonads

paCO$_2$ Partial pressure of carbon dioxide in the arterial blood

paO$_2$ Partial pressure of oxygen in the arterial blood

paediatrician A doctor specialising in the care of infants and children. Some paediatricians specialise in caring for the newborn–neonatologists

paracervical block Process by which the area on each side of the cervix is anaesthetised by the injection of a local anaesthetic to relieve the pain of the first stage of labour.

parentcraft classes A series of meetings held in pregnancy to discuss relevant issues, e.g. preparation for labour and the arrival of the baby. These may be held in the maternity unit, in community clinics or privately by such groups as the National Childbirth Trust

parity Refers to the number of times a woman has given birth to a baby

pelvic brim Inlet of the pelvis

pentazocine (Fortral) Analgesic prescribed for moderate to severe pain

perinatal mortality rate The number of stillbirths plus newborn deaths occurring during the first week of life per 1000 total births

perineal Pertaining to the perineum – an area of fibrous tissue and muscle between the vaginal and anal canals

pethidine An analgesic used to relieve the pain of labour

placenta The afterbirth

progesterone A hormone produced by the corpus

luteum and placenta in pregnancy

prolonged labour Labour which extends beyond the usual time span, i.e. 18 hours for a primigravida and 12 hours for a multigravida when the uterus is contracting properly.

prolonged rupture of membranes When the fetal sac has broken spontaneously resulting in the release of amniotic fluid but with no accompanying uterine contractions within 24 hours

prospective research Events yet to happen are investigated as opposed to retrospective research which depends on information already received

prostaglandins A group of substances used to soften the neck of the uterus and induce labour

psychiatric Relating to mental disorders

psychoprophylaxis One of the alternative methods of pain relief in labour. Principles are to allay anxiety, encourage relaxation, provide distraction and encourage a positive attitude

pudendal block Process by which pudendal nerves are anaesthetised by the injection of a local anaesthetic to relieve the discomfort of the second stage of labour

registrar A doctor who has practised as a Senior House Officer for at least two years and is now continuing in his or her chosen specialty. During this post he or she will obtain a higher diploma as a Member of the Royal College of Obstetricians and Gynaecologists

relaxation exercises Exercises practised in pregnancy to reduce tension in preparation for coping with the contractions during labour

respiratory Pertaining to breathing

scopolamine (Hyoscine) Drug used in conjunction with analgesic, e.g. Omnopon, when antisecretory effects are desired

senior house officer A doctor who has completed a year of general medical surgical training after qualification and has now joined a specialty, e.g. obstetrics

senior registrar A doctor who has been promoted from registrar level where he/she worked for 3 or 4 years. Most become consultants in 3–4 years

shoulder presentation This arises if the fetus is lying obliquely when labour starts. The fetal shoulder descends into the maternal pelvis and labour becomes obstructed

spontaneous delivery Childbirth which occurs naturally without stimulation and needing no instrumental aid

stillbirth A baby born dead after the 28th week of pregnancy. From October 1992 this has become 24 weeks

syntocinon A drug given to stimulate contractions of the uterus and so induce or accelerate labour

TENS (Transcutaneous electrical nerve stimulation) A method of pain relief in labour. Electrodes are placed on the skin to produce a pulsed electrical current which interrupts pain transmission and stimulates the production of endogenous opiates

tidal volume The amount of air inhaled and exhaled during ventilation

trichlorethylene (trilene) An inhalational analgesia no longer approved for use by midwives

t-test Test to compare two groups of measurements. The two sets of data must come from populations that are normal and have the same amount of variance

uterus Muscular pelvic organ the function of which is to contain and sustain the fetus during pregnancy and expel the baby during labour

vacuum extraction A method of delivering the baby by applying suction to a cup applied to the baby's head. The scalp is then drawn gently into the cap by the use of the vacuum and the baby is guided through the birth canal with the assistance of traction

vagina Canal which runs from the cervix to the exterior orifice

ventilation Process by which gases are moved in and out of the lungs artificially

version Obstetric procedure in which a fetus presenting feet first is turned and delivered head first

vertex An area of the baby's head which presents first at delivery when the attitude is one good flexion, i.e. normal presentation

vulva External female genital organs

Appendix – The Questionnaires

The following pages reproduce the questionnaires used for the National Birthday Trust Survey 1990.

Branch 1 was sent to all units before the survey started.

Branch 2A was given to the midwives actually at delivery. **Branch 2B** was given by the midwife to the woman and her partner to fill in.

Branch 3 was sent by post to 10% of these women after delivery for filling in at home.

DELIVERY UNIT CODE

INFORMATION ABOUT DELIVERY UNIT

PAIN RELIEF IN CHILDBIRTH
(Branch 1)

A CONFIDENTIAL ENQUIRY
CONDUCTED BY

THE NATIONAL BIRTHDAY TRUST
1990

HOSPITAL NAME _____

ADDRESS _____

_____

REGION/
HEALTH BOARD _____

Please return completed forms to:
ANN WRAIGHT, Survey Co-ordinator
Department of Obstetrics & Gynaecology
St George's Hospital Medical School
Cranmer Terrace
London SW17 0RE

NOTES FOR GUIDANCE

Branch 1 of the Survey Questionnaire has been designed to provide a profile of your delivery suite. The information is needed so that facilities and policies can be related to the pain relief achieved by women in labour.

The questions should be answered by a senior midwife when the survey has been completed. Please return it to us using the Freepost label enclosed.

The information will be entirely confidential and it must be stressed that there will be no means of identifying units. A survey number will be given to the form as soon as it reaches us and identifying details will be removed. This will be done even before coding and thereafter the form will be identified by the survey number only.

Definitions

Page 1 — The last available year should be 1989 if possible. Most units now collect statistical data from April to March so therefore the year relates to 1st April 1989 to 31st March 1990; others still collect from January to December, therefore the year relates to 1st January to 31st December 1989. Please indicate which you use in box 2.

Perinatal Mortality Rate (PMR)

If your unit accepts in utero transfers, please differentiate between the PMR which includes these from the rate which does not.

If you have not admitted any in utero transfers, record your PMR in the ''PMR excluding'' column.

The PMR should include only babies born in your unit.

We would like to emphasise that this is a National survey and not an assessment of your individual unit. Thank you for the time you have given to help us gather the data.

ANN WRAIGHT

GEOFFREY CHAMBERLAIN

NATIONAL BIRTHDAY TRUST

DELIVERY UNIT CODE [   ]

BACKGROUND INFORMATION ABOUT YOUR UNIT

1

TYPE OF UNIT:

	Please tick one only
NHS Consultant Unit	☐ 1
Combined GP and Consultant Unit	☐ 2
Combined Consultant Unit and Private Unit	☐ 3
General Practitioner Unit	
—separate in NHS hospital, but with Consultant cover	☐ 4
—separate in NHS hospital, without Consultant cover	☐ 5
—isolated	☐ 6
Private Unit in NHS hospital	☐ 7
Armed Services	☐ 8
Private Hospital	☐ 9
Other—please specify:	☐ 10

2

PLEASE COMPLETE THE FOLLOWING DETAILS FOR THE LAST AVAILABLE YEAR
(see notes for guidance)

Number of deliveries: ☐☐☐☐

Number of babies born <2500g ☐☐☐

Number of Caesarean sections: ☐☐☐

In utero transfers

—None ☐

—No. of mothers transferred from your Unit (OUT): ☐☐☐

—No. of mothers transferred into your Unit (IN): ☐☐☐

Perinatal Mortality Rate per 1000 births
(excluding in utero transfers) ☐☐☐

Perinatal Mortality Rate per 1000 births
(including in utero transfers) ☐☐☐

Please record the statistical year to which these figures relate _____

3 No. of births (including home confinement within your area) which took place on the week of the survey ☐☐☐

4 When the woman requests analgesia which professional advises the woman?

PLEASE TICK ANY THAT APPLY

Obstetrician	1 ☐
Midwife	2 ☐
Anaesthetist	3 ☐
Other	4 ☐
Specify _____	

5	Which analgesic methods are available? (PLEASE TICK ANY THAT APPLY)		
		Pethidine	1 ☐
		$N_2O + O_2$	2 ☐
		Epidural	3 ☐
		Other (pharmacological method)	4 ☐
		Specify _____	
		Hypnosis	5 ☐
		Acupuncture	6 ☐
		Relaxation & Breathing	7 ☐
		TENS	8 ☐
		Other (non-pharmacological method)	9 ☐
		Specify _____	

6	If epidural analgesia is available is it		
		On medical indication?	1 ☐
		In daytime only?	2 ☐
		For the whole 24 hours?	3 ☐

7	Is it started by		
		Anaesthetist?	1 ☐
		Obstetrician?	2 ☐

8	Who gives top-up injections or refills syringe pumps?		
		Anaesthetist	1 ☐
		Midwife	2 ☐
		Obstetrician	3 ☐
		General Practitioner	4 ☐
		Other	5 ☐
		Specify _____	

STAFFING

Please record the number of Anaesthetists (or other Doctors who give anaesthetics) who are on duty to provide care for women in the delivery area <u>on the first day of the survey.</u>

9	NHS equivalent status of doctors	Available for delivery area		
		On duty in the hospital premises	Not in the hospital but on call within 20 mins	>20 mins
		1	2	3
	Consultant	☐ 1	☐ 1	☐ 1
	Senior Registrar	☐ 2	☐ 2	☐ 2
	Associate Specialist	☐ 3	☐ 3	☐ 3
	Registrar	☐ 4	☐ 4	☐ 4
	Clinical assistant	☐ 5	☐ 5	☐ 5
	G.P.	☐ 6	☐ 6	☐ 6
	S.H.O.	☐ 7	☐ 7	☐ 7
	Other	☐ 8	☐ 8	☐ 8
	Specify _____			

NOTES FOR GUIDANCE

The aim of this enquiry is to obtain an assessment of *EVERY* delivery (vaginal and Caesarean section) which takes place in the U.K. from *0900 25.06.90 until 0859 02.07.90.* All the information requested relates to the woman's pain control in labour (with or without analgesia) so that comparisons can be made between the professionals' and the consumers' views.

Each section needs to be completed by the different people involved but not all questions/sections will be applicable to every labour.

    White —Midwife
    Blue   —Obstetrician/G.P. (Only if involved in the labour sufficiently to assess effectiveness of
                    pain relief.)
    Orange—Anaesthetist (Only if involved in the labour sufficiently to assess effectiveness of pain
                    relief.)
    Yellow —Paediatrician
    Pink   —Woman
    Green —Husband/Partner/Companion

Please try to complete the forms even if the baby is stillborn, as we need information about these mothers, however, we leave it to your descretion to omit questions if they would cause hurt to the parents.

Each person is asked to give his/her own assessment of the woman's pain relief. This obviously needs to be done *INDEPENDENTLY SO THAT THE ANSWERS ARE UNBIASED.* Remember that this is a National Survey and not an assessment of any one professional group or individual unit. The information is entirely confidential so there will be no means of identifying people or hospitals. A survey number will be given to the form while personal and geographical details removed.

Please hand over the questionnaire, if incomplete, to the midwife who is taking over the woman's care. Please return the questionnaires, when completed, to the Senior Midwife who is co-ordinating the collection in your unit.

Remember that the *more complete the questionnaires, the more valid the findings.* We appreciate the time this consumes and thank you for your commitment to this National enquiry.

ANN WRAIGHT

GEOFFREY CHAMBERLAIN

National Birthday Trust

THE MIDWIFE

(a) Pages 1-4

—All the details required on these pages can be obtained from the woman's notes following delivery.

—Please give details as precisely as possible of the occupation, i.e., the job she/he does rather than that of the employing company. If unemployed, give last employment. If not known, write N/K.

—If this is a multiple pregnancy, a separate form should be completed for each delivery and each baby (i.e., pages 2, 4 and 8). Your Senior Midwife will have a stock of these. Please identify each page with the appropriate survey number.

—Estimated gestation should be the most accurate known, i.e., by ultrasound scan if that has been done and if necessary any revised calculation of stage of gestation.

—The commencement of labour = the onset of regular, rhythmic uterine contractions accompanied by progressive dilatation of the cervical os.

(b) Page 5

—An interpreter may be a member of the woman's family, a member of staff or anyone who facilitates language communication.

—An assessment of the woman's pain control by the midwife who was most involved with the labour. All methods used should be assessed, e.g., bath, massage, relaxation exercises as well as drugs used for local and general anaesthesia.

—This assessment needs to be made as soon as possible after delivery to make it valid.

BRANCH 2A

DELIVERY UNIT CODE ☐

SURVEY NO. ☐

1. DESCRIPTIVE DATA OF THE WOMAN
PLEASE TICK ONE ONLY UNLESS OTHERWISE INSTRUCTED

1 | **Ethnic Origin:** White | ☐ 1
| Black—Caribbean | ☐ 2
| Black—African | ☐ 3
| Black—Other | ☐ 4
| Indian | ☐ 5
| Pakistani | ☐ 6
| Bangladeshi | ☐ 7
| Chinese | ☐ 8
| Other Asian | ☐ 9
| Any other ethnic group | ☐ 10

2 | **Age** | ☐☐ years

3 | **At booking, was the woman:**
| Single | ☐ 1
| Married | ☐ 2
| Separated | ☐ 3
| Divorced | ☐ 4
| Widowed | ☐ 5

4 | **In this pregnancy, was the woman:**
| Supported | ☐ 1
| Unsupported | ☐ 2

5 | **Occupation** (See notes of Guidance)

WOMAN'S PRESENT/LAST JOB	HUSBAND'S/PARTNER'S PRESENT/LAST JOB

6 | **Past obstetrical history** (Tick any that apply)
| Number of Previous Live Births | ☐ 1
| Number of Previous Still Births | ☐ 2
| Number of Early Pregnancy Losses | ☐ 3
| Number of Neonatal Deaths | ☐ 4

2. CARE IN LABOUR

7 | WERE ANY OF THE FOLLOWING COMPLICATIONS PRESENT AT THE ONSET OF LABOUR? (Tick any that apply)
| Hypertensive disease | ☐ 1
| Neurological disease | ☐ 2
| Cardiac disease | ☐ 3
| Diabetes | ☐ 4
| Antepartum haemorrhage | ☐ 5
| Psychiatric disorders | ☐ 6
| Intrauterine Growth Retardation | ☐ 7
| Prolonged rupture of membranes | ☐ 8
| Other Specify:_____ | ☐

8 | **Estimated gestation** | ☐☐
| (See notes of Guidance) | Weeks

9 | **Was the delivery:**
| Single | ☐ 1
| Twin | ☐ 2
| Other | ☐ 3
| (If multiple delivery, please complete two or more forms as necessary, ie, pages 2, 4, and 8) |

10 | **Presentation of Fetus at Onset of Labour**

Vertex ☐ 1
Breech ☐ 2
Face ☐ 3
Brow ☐ 4
Shoulder ☐ 5
Compound ☐ 6

11 | **If labour took place, did it start:**
Spontaneously ☐ 1
Induced ☐ 2

12 | **If Induced or Augmented what methods were used:**
(Tick any that apply)
Prostaglandins ☐ 1
Syntocinon ☐ 2
A.R.M. ☐ 3
Other ☐ 4
INDICATION FOR INDUCTION_____

13 | **If A.R.M., Time of Procedure**
HOURS ☐☐ MINUTES ☐☐

14 | (See notes of guidance)
DAY MONTH HOURS MINUTES
Date and time of baby's birth _____/_____ ☐☐ ☐☐
1st stage of labour ☐☐ ☐☐
2nd stage of labour ☐☐ ☐☐
3rd stage of labour ☐☐ ☐☐

15 | **Method of Delivery:**
Spontaneous: Cephalic Anterior ☐ 1
Cephalic Posterior ☐ 2
Breech ☐ 3
Face ☐ 4
Assisted: Forceps:
Cephalic — traction only ☐ 5
— with rotation ☐ 6
Breech ☐ 7
Vacuum Extraction ☐ 8
IF DELIVERY WAS BY CAESAREAN SECTION, WAS IT:
Planned — Before labour ☐ 9
Unplanned — Before labour ☐ 10
Planned — In labour ☐ 11
Unplanned — In labour ☐ 12

16 | Indications for assisted delivery _____

17 | Indications for Caesarean section _____

18 | **Was the placenta removed manually?**
YES ☐
NO ☐

19 | In the following three tables, please list the alternative methods and the drugs the woman used to control her pain.
NB. This should include *all 3 stages of labour.*
ALTERNATIVE METHODS, e.g., MASSAGE, TENS

			1	2	3	4	5
METHOD	DECIDED BY WHOM	LENGTH OF TIME USED	AT WHAT STAGE OF LABOUR 1ST			2ND	3RD
			Early	Middle	Late		

20 | Inhalation Analgesia, e.g. $N_2O + O_2$ (Entonox)

			1	2	3	4	5
METHOD	DECIDED BY WHOM	LENGTH OF TIME USED	AT WHAT STAGE OF LABOUR 1ST			2ND	3RD
			Early	Middle	Late		

21 | Drugs, e.g. Marcain, Lignocaine Pethidine

			1	2	3	4	5
METHOD	DECIDED BY WHOM	TOTAL DOSE	AT WHAT STAGE OF LABOUR 1ST			2ND	3RD
			Early	Middle	Late		

22 | If epidural or spinal anaesthesia used:

HOURS   MINUTES

—Time inserted

—Number of attempts

—Grade of anaesthetist

23 | Was a general anaesthetic given?   YES ☐   NO ☐

3. THE BABY

24	**Was the baby born:**	LIVE ☐ 1
		DEAD ☐ 2

| 25 | **Birth weight** | ☐ ☐ ☐ ☐ g |

26	**Apgar score** —at 1 minute	1 ☐ ☐
	—at 5 minutes	2 ☐ ☐
	—at 10 minutes	3 ☐ ☐

27	**Was the baby resuscitated?**	YES ☐
		NO ☐

28	**If Yes:** —facial oxygen	1 ☐
	—bag and mask ventilation	2 ☐
	—endotracheal tube ventilation	3 ☐
	Artificial ventilation started (minutes after birth)	☐ ☐
	First spontaneous breath (minutes after birth)	☐ ☐
	Artificial ventilation stopped (if still in Labour Ward, minutes after birth)	☐ ☐

29	**Who resuscitated the baby initially?**	
	Midwife	1 ☐
	Paediatrician	2 ☐
	Other	3 ☐
	Specify: _____	
	N/A	4 ☐

30	**Were drugs used in resuscitation**	YES 1 ☐
		NO 2 ☐
		N/A 3 ☐
	If Yes: Naloxone	YES ☐
		NO ☐
		N/A ☐
	If Naloxone was used, was it given	I.V. 1 ☐
		I.M. 2 ☐
		N/A 3 ☐
	—Others	YES ☐
		NO ☐
	Specify: _____	

31	**Was the baby admitted to the neonatal unit?**	YES ☐
		NO ☐

THANK YOU FOR COMPLETING THIS QUESTIONNAIRE SO FAR.
THE FOLLOWING SECTIONS NOW NEED TO BE DONE BY THE VARIOUS PEOPLE INVOLVED
IN THE LABOUR.

4. MIDWIFE WHO WAS MOST INVOLVED WITH THIS LABOUR

PLEASE TICK APPROPRIATE BOXES

1   **Was an interpreter necessary for communication with the woman?**

YES ☐
NO ☐

2   **If yes, was the interpreter used?**

YES ☐
NO ☐

3   **If the woman used any method of pain relief during labour:**

PLEASE INDICATE THE DEGREE OF EFFECT OF EACH METHOD AND ANY COMPLICATION
NOTED FOR EACH METHOD USED. (Include alternative methods)

BEST EFFECT AT TIME USED
1   2   3   4

METHOD	Very good	Good	Poor	No use	Complication

4   **Was there any difficulty in obtaining Analgesia/Anaesthesia?**

YES ☐
NO ☐

5   **Do you attribute these difficulties to any factors?**

YES ☐ 1
NO ☐ 2
N/A ☐ 3

IF YES: PLEASE SPECIFY: _____

: _____

6   **What was the time interval between requesting an epidural and its completion?**

HOURS   MINUTES
☐ ☐   ☐ ☐

7   **How many years have you practised as a midwife?** _____

8   **Questionnaire completed:**   DATE .... / .... / ....
TIME: ☐ ☐ ☐ ☐

THANK YOU FOR COMPLETING THIS QUESTIONNAIRE. PLEASE USE THE SPACE BELOW IF YOU WISH
TO ADD FURTHER COMMENTS.

5. THE OBSTETRICIAN OR GENERAL PRACTITIONER WHO WAS INVOLVED WITH THIS LABOUR/PRESENT AT DELIVERY

PLEASE TICK APPROPRIATE BOXES

| 1 | Did you make any assessment of the effect of analgesics? | | | | | YES ☐ NO ☐ |

2   Please indicate the degree of effect of each method and any complication noted for each method used. (Include alternative methods.)

BEST EFFECT AT TIME USED
1   2   3   4

METHOD	Very good	Good	Poor	No use	Complication

| 3 | Was there any difficulty in getting Analgesia/Anaesthesia? | YES ☐ NO ☐ |

| 4 | Do you attribute these difficulties to any factors? | YES ☐ NO ☐ |

If Yes: Please specify: _____

_____

| 5 | Grade of Doctor completing form: |

| 6 | Questionnaire completed: | DATE.........../.........../............. TIME: ☐ ☐ ☐ ☐ |

THANK YOU FOR ANSWERING THESE QUESTIONS. PLEASE USE THE SPACE BELOW IF YOU WISH TO ADD FURTHER COMMENTS.

6. ANAESTHETIST OR OTHER DOCTOR GIVING THE ANAESTHETIC INVOLVED IN THE CASE/ PRESENT AT DELIVERY:

PLEASE TICK APPROPRIATE BOXES

1. Did you make any assessment of the effect of analgesia?　　　YES ☐　NO ☐

2. Please indicate the degree of effect of each method and any complication noted for each method used. (Include alternative methods.)

BEST EFFECT AT TIME USED
1　2　3　4

METHOD	Very good	Good	Poor	No use	Complication

3. Was there any difficulty in achieving effective Analgesia/Anaesthesia?　　YES ☐　NO ☐

4. Do you attribute these difficulties to any factors?　　YES ☐　NO ☐

   If yes: Please specify: _____

5. What was the time interval between receiving the request for epidural and completing the procedure?　　HOURS ☐☐　MINUTES ☐☐

6. Grade of anaesthetist completing form: _____

7. Questionnaire completed:　DATE:........./........./..........　TIME: ☐☐☐☐

THANK YOU FOR ANSWERING THESE QUESTIONS. PLEASE USE THE SPACE BELOW IF YOU WISH TO ADD ANY FURTHER COMMENTS.

7. PAEDIATRICIAN OR OTHER PROFESSIONAL WHO EXAMINES THE BABY WITHIN 24 HOURS

PLEASE TICK APPROPRIATE BOX

1   Status of paediatrician?

Senior House Officer ☐ 1
Registrar ☐ 2
Consultant ☐ 3

2   If not a paediatrician, who examined the baby?

Obstetrician ☐ 1
General Practitioner ☐ 2
Midwife ☐ 3
Other ☐ 4
Specify: _____

3   Age of baby?   Hours: ☐☐

4   Were any of the following conditions reported to you or noted at examination?

	REPORTED	NOTED
Hypothermia	☐ 1	☐ 1
Hypoglycaemia	☐ 2	☐ 2
Excessively sleepy	☐ 3	☐ 3
Hypotonia	☐ 4	☐ 4
Poor feeding	☐ 5	☐ 5
Apnoea	☐ 6	☐ 6
Other respiratory problems	☐ 7	☐ 7
Difficult to console	☐ 8	☐ 8
Other conditions likely to be due to analgesia in labour or following delivery	☐ 9	☐ 9

Specify: _____

5   Is there any medical diagnosis to account for above abnormality (ies)?   YES ☐   NO ☐

If Yes: Specify: _____

THANK YOU FOR ANSWERING THESE QUESTIONS. PLEASE USE THE SPACE BELOW IF YOU WISH TO ADD ANY FURTHER COMMENTS.

8. THIS SECTION TO BE COMPLETED BY THE *WOMAN* HERSELF

1 | **Where did you get your information about pain relief in labour?** (Tick any that apply)

Books	☐ 1
Magazines	☐ 2
Newspapers	☐ 3
TV/Radio	☐ 4
Family	☐ 5
Friends/Other women	☐ 6
Antenatal classes	☐ 7
Midwives	☐ 8
Doctors	☐ 9
Previous experience of labour	☐ 10
Other	☐ 11
Specify: _____	

2 | **Did you go to any antenatal or parentcraft classes?** YES ☐ NO ☐

3 | **What sort of classes were they?** (Tick any that apply)

Hospital	☐ 1
Health Centre or other clinic	☐ 2
National Childbirth Trust	☐ 3
Other	☐ 4
Specify: _____	

4 | **Which methods of pain relief did you plan to use and then actually used in your labour?**

TICK ANY THAT APPLY

	Planned to use	Used
None	☐ 1	☐ 1
Pethidine	☐ 2	☐ 2
Gas—Nitrous Oxide + Oxygen	☐ 3	☐ 3
Epidural	☐ 4	☐ 4
Relaxation and Breathing	☐ 5	☐ 5
Massage	☐ 6	☐ 6
TENS	☐ 7	☐ 7
Other	☐ 8	☐ 8
Specify: _____		

IF YOU DID NOT EXPERIENCE LABOUR AT ALL, PLEASE MOVE ON TO QUESTION 13.

5 | **Who was with you during labour *before* you came into hospital?** (Tick any that apply)

		For how long?
Does not apply	☐ 1	
Alone	☐ 2	Hours: ☐ ☐
Husband/Partner	☐ 3	Hours: ☐ ☐
Other family	☐ 4	Hours: ☐ ☐
Midwife	☐ 5	Hours: ☐ ☐
GP	☐ 6	Hours: ☐ ☐
Other	☐ 7	Hours: ☐ ☐
Specify: _____		

6 | **Who was with you during labour *after* you came into hospital?** (Tick any that apply)

		For how long?
Does not apply	☐ 1	
Alone	☐ 2	Hours: ☐ ☐
Husband/Partner	☐ 3	Hours: ☐ ☐
Other family	☐ 4	Hours: ☐ ☐
Midwife	☐ 5	Hours: ☐ ☐
GP	☐ 6	Hours: ☐ ☐
Other	☐ 7	Hours: ☐ ☐
Specify: _____		

7 During labour, were there times when you were:

(Tick all that apply)
IF YES, AT WHAT STAGE OF LABOUR

		1 EARLY	2 MIDDLE	3 LATE
PAIN FREE?	YES ☐ NO ☐	☐	☐	☐
IN MILD PAIN?	YES ☐ NO ☐	☐	☐	☐
IN SEVERE BUT BEARABLE PAIN?	YES ☐ NO ☐	☐	☐	☐
IN UNBEARABLE PAIN?	YES ☐ NO ☐	☐	☐	☐

8 What do you think was:

(a) MOST HELPFUL IN RELIEVING PAIN?
Specify: _____

(b) MOST UNHELPFUL IN RELIEVING PAIN?
Specify: _____

9 Were you able to relax?   YES ☐   NO ☐

If yes, what helped you to do that and at what stage of labour? (Tick all that apply)

FACTOR WHICH HELPED YOU RELAX	EARLY STAGE	MIDDLE STAGE	LATE STAGE

10 If no, what interfered with relaxation (apart from the pain)?

Restricted to bed	1	☐
Unfamiliar surroundings	2	☐
Strangers	3	☐
Noise	4	☐
Monitor	5	☐
Bright lights	6	☐
Too many people	7	☐
Given conflicting advice	8	☐
Anxiety	9	☐
Other	10	☐

Specify: _____

11 Was there a bath/shower available for your use to relieve pain in labour?

YES ☐
NO ☐

12 Did you use it?   YES ☐   NO ☐

13 Please indicate the degree of effect of each method of pain control you used. (Include anything you used, e.g., massage, relaxation, general anaesthetic)

METHOD	1 VERY GOOD	2 GOOD	3 POOR	4 NO USE	1 GIVEN AT RIGHT TIME	2 GIVEN TOO EARLY	3 GIVEN TOO LATE	4 DON'T KNOW

IF YOU DID NOT EXPERIENCE LABOUR, PLEASE MOVE ON TO QUESTION 20

14 **How much did you feel you were free to choose pain relief?** (Tick one only)

Very free	⊔ 1
Quite free	⊔ 2
Not very free	⊔ 3
Not at all free	⊔ 4

15 **Who suggested starting pain relief?** (Tick one only)

You	⊔ 1
Your Partner or Companion	⊔ 2
Obstetrician	⊔ 3
Midwife	⊔ 4
Anaesthetist	⊔ 5
Other	⊔ 6

Specify: _____

16 **Were you cared for by the same midwife only throughout your whole labour?**

YES ⊔

NO ⊔

If, no, how many midwives looked after you? ⊔

17 **If you had a forceps or vacuum delivery, was it painful?**   YES ⊔   NO ⊔

IF IT WAS PAINFUL, WAS IT

—Mild Pain?	⊔ 1
—Severe but bearable?	⊔ 2
—Unbearable?	⊔ 3
—N/A?	⊔ 4

18 **Did you have stitches? (Omit this question if you had a Caesarean section)**

YES ⊔

NO ⊔

If yes, what form of pain relief did you have for their insertion?

None	⊔ 1
Gas—Nitrous Oxide + Oxygen	⊔ 2
Injection	⊔ 3
Epidural	⊔ 4
Don't know	⊔ 5

Other—Specify: _____

19 **What methods of pain relief would you choose or not choose if you have another baby?** (Tick more than one if you want to)

	CHOOSE 1	WOULD NOT CHOOSE 2	DON'T KNOW 3
Pethidine	⊔	⊔	⊔
Gas—Nitrous Oxide + Oxygen	⊔	⊔	⊔
Epidural or similar	⊔	⊔	⊔
Relaxation and Breathing	⊔	⊔	⊔
Massage	⊔	⊔	⊔
TENS	⊔	⊔	⊔
Other	⊔	⊔	⊔

Specify: _____

Give reasons: _____

IF YOU HAD A CAESAREAN SECTION (WHETHER YOU EXPERIENCED SOME LABOUR OR NONE AT ALL) PLEASE ANSWER THE FOLLOWING 3 QUESTIONS

20 **What type of anaesthetic were you given?** (Tick any that apply)

Epidural ☐ 1
General Anaesthetic ☐ 2
Other ☐ 3

21 **Who discussed the method of choice with you?** (Tick one only)

Anaesthetist ☐ 1
Obstetrician ☐ 2
GP ☐ 3
Midwife ☐ 4
No one ☐ 5
Other ☐ 6
Specify: _____

22 **Under general anaesthetic were you aware of any feelings or sounds during the operation?** (Tick any that apply)

Pain ☐ 1
Touch ☐ 2
People ☐ 3
Other ☐ 4
Specify: _____

EVERYONE SHOULD ANSWER THE LAST THREE QUESTIONS

23 **Did you notice any side effects of the pain relief on yourself?**

YES   NO   DON'T KNOW
1   2   3
☐   ☐   ☐
If Yes: What were these? ____

24 **Did you think the method of pain relief affected the baby?**

YES   NO   DON'T KNOW
1   2   3
☐   ☐   ☐
If Yes: In what way? _____

25 **Is there any information about pain relief you now wish you had known?**

YES ☐
NO ☐
If Yes: Specify: _____
_____

26 Date Completed: Date ..../......./.......
Time ☐ ☐ ☐ ☐

THANK YOU FOR ANSWERING ALL THESE QUESTIONS. PLEASE USE THE SPACE BELOW TO ADD ANY FURTHER COMMENTS.

27 **May we send you a follow-up questionnaire in 6 weeks' time?**

YES ☐
NO ☐

If yes, please record the address you will be residing at, on the tear off slip below.

9. THIS SECTION TO BE COMPLETED BY THE HUSBAND/PARTNER OR COMPANION PRESENT IN LABOUR

1 **Where did you get your information about pain relief in labour?** (Tick any that apply)

Books	1
Magazines	2
Newspapers	3
TV/Radio	4
Family	5
Your Partner	6
Friends	7
Antenatal classes	8
Midwives	9
Doctors	10
Your experience of partner's previous labour(s)	11
Other	12

Specify: _____

2 **Did you go to antenatal or parentcraft classes**   YES ☐   NO ☐

3 **When she was in labour, or in the theatre, were you with her** (Tick one only)

None of the time?	1
Some of the time?	2
All the time?	3

IF THE BABY WAS BORN BY CAESAREAN SECTION PLEASE MOVE ON TO QUESTION 8

4 **During her labour, were there times when she was:**

(Tick all that apply)
IF YES, AT WHAT STAGE OF LABOUR

			1 EARLY	2 MIDDLE	3 LATE
PAIN FREE?	YES ☐		☐	☐	☐
	NO ☐				
IN MILD PAIN?	YES ☐		☐	☐	☐
	NO ☐				
IN SEVERE BUT BEARABLE PAIN?	YES ☐		☐	☐	☐
	NO ☐				
IN UNBEARABLE PAIN?	YES ☐		☐	☐	☐
	NO ☐				

5 **What do you think was**

(a) Most helpful in avoiding/relieving pain?
Specify: _____

(b) Most unhelpful in relieving pain?
Specify: _____

6 If your partner used any method of pain relief during labour:
Please indicate the degree of effect of each method of pain control your partner used, eg, massage, relaxation, general anaesthetic

	1	2	3	4	1	2	3	4
METHOD	VERY GOOD	GOOD	POOR	NO USE	GIVEN AT RIGHT TIME	GIVEN TOO EARLY	GIVEN TOO LATE	DON'T KNOW

7 To what extent do you think you were able to help her with pain? (Tick one only)

As much as I liked	☐	1
To quite an extent	☐	2
Not at all	☐	3
Don't know	☐	4

8 Is there any information about pain relief you now wish you had known?

YES ☐
NO ☐

If Yes, What? _____
_____

9 Date: completed: Date............../.............../..............
Time   ☐ ☐ ☐ ☐

THANK YOU FOR ANSWERING THESE QUESTIONS. PLEASE USE THE SPACE BELOW TO ADD ANY FURTHER COMMENTS.

PAIN RELIEF IN LABOUR SURVEY

You may remember that some weeks ago, just after you had given birth to your baby, you completed a questionnaire on your pain relief in labour. We would be grateful if you would now answer a few more questions, as we would like to compare the feelings women have about this some weeks after birth with those they had soon after delivery.

The general aim of the survey is to improve the care given to mothers and babies. To do that, we need suggestions and comments from mothers, like yourself, who have recently experienced labour.

We would like to stress that the answers you give will be entirely confidential. Your name does not appear on the survey itself, and no mention about the results of the survey will be available to anyone who was involved in your care. Your hospital is not involved in this part of the survey.

We are indebted to you for the help you are giving us. You will find enclosed a Business Reply label (Freepost) to use with the original envelope. When you have answered all the questions, please replace the form in the envelope, seal it and return it to us within two weeks.

Thank you again for participating in this study.

Professor G. Chamberlain
DIRECTOR

Mrs Ann Wraight
CO-ORDINATOR

FOR EACH QUESTION, PLEASE CIRCLE <u>ONE NUMBER ONLY.</u>
PLEASE FEEL FREE TO ADD NOTES, COMMENTS, EXPLANATIONS.
WE HAVE LEFT SPACE AT THE END FOR YOU TO WRITE FURTHER NOTES
IF YOU WISH.

Your feelings about the birth now.

1.
On the whole, did you enjoy the birth of your baby?	1 Yes
	2 No
	3 Other _____
	8 Don't know

2.
How much in control of your labour did you feel?	1 Completely in control
	2 Quite in control
	3 Not very in control
	4 Not at all in control
	5 Other _____
	8 Don't know

3.
How much in control of the delivery of your baby did you feel?	1 Completely in control
	2 Quite in control
	3 Not very in control
	4 Not at all in control
	5 Other _____
	8 Don't know

4.
How much pain would you say you felt during the labour?	1 A great deal, unbearable
	2 A great deal, bearable
	3 Some pain
	4 Very little pain
	5 No pain at all because of effective pain relief
	6 No pain at all without any pain relief
	7 Other _____
	8 Don't know

5. How much pain would you say you felt during the delivery of your baby?

1 A great deal, unbearable
2 A great deal, bearable
3 Some pain
4 Very little pain
5 No pain at all because of effective pain relief
6 No pain at all without any pain relief
7 Other _____
8 Don't know

6. How do you feel about the care you received from the midwives at the birth?

1 Very satisfied
2 Satisfied
3 Dissatisfied
4 Very dissatisfied
8 Don't know

7. How do you feel about the care you received from the doctors at the birth?

1 Very satisfied
2 Satisfied
3 Dissatisfied
4 Very dissatisfied
8 Don't know

8. How do you feel now overall about the pain relief you had during labour and delivery?

1 Very satisfied
2 Satisfied
3 Dissatisfied
4 Very dissatisfied
8 Don't know

9. Do you feel you had pain relief at the right time?

1 Yes
2 No, too early
3 No, too late
4 Other _____
8 Don't know

10. How much do you feel now you were able to choose the kind of pain relief you had?

1 Very free
2 Quite free
3 Not very free
4 Not at all free

11. Looking back on it now, is there any information you would like to have had about pain relief which you were not given?

1 Yes
2 No
8 Don't know

If yes, please specify: _____

_____

12. What methods of pain relief would you choose (or not choose) if you had another baby? (Please circle all appropriate numbers.)

	1 Choose	2 Not choose	8 Don't know
Pethidine	1	1	1
Gas and O_2 (Entonox)	2	2	2
Epidural	3	3	3
Breathing exercises	4	4	4
Massage	5	5	5
TENS	6	6	6
None	7	7	7
Other	8	8	8

Specify_____

13. If you had another baby would you choose to have it in the same place as this one?

1 Yes
2 No
3 Not sure
8 Don't know

14. Did the pain relief you had at the birth affect the way you felt afterwards, while you were in hospital?

1 Yes
2 No
3 Other _____
8 Don't know

If yes, please explain _____

_____

15. Did you feel the pain relief you had at
the birth has in any way affected you
since you came home from hospital?

1 Yes
2 No
3 Other _____
8 Don't know

If yes, please explain _____

_____

16. Do you think the pain relief you had
affected the baby afterwards?

1 Yes
2 No
3 Other _____
8 Don't know

If yes, please explain _____

_____

17. Do you feel it affected the baby's
feeding in any way?

1 Yes
2 No
3 Other _____
8 Don't know

If yes, please explain _____

_____

Your feelings since the birth and about looking after the baby.

18. Since the birth how have you felt physically?

1 Very well
2 Well
3 Not very well
4 Not at all well
8 Don't know

19. Have you had any of these problems as a result of the birth? (Please circle all appropriate numbers.)

	1 A lot	2 A little	3 None
Discomfort caused by stitches	1	1	1
Passing water when you don't want to	2	2	2
Need to pass water frequently	3	3	3
Piles	4	4	4
Varicose veins	5	5	5
Breast abscess	6	6	6
Cracked nipples	7	7	7
Engorgement of breasts	8	8	8
Problems related to Caesarean birth	9	9	9
If yes, please specify			
Other physical problems	10	10	10
If yes, please specify			

20. Since the birth how have you felt in yourself?

1 Very happy
2 Happy
3 Quite depressed
4 Very depressed
5 Other _____
8 Don't know

21. How confident do you feel as a mother?

1 Very confident about everything
2 Confident about most things
3 Not very confident
4 Not at all confident
5 Other _____
8 Don't know

22. How would you describe your baby's temperament?
1 Generally happy
2 Sometimes happy, sometimes miserable
3 Generally difficult
4 Other _____
8 Don't know

23. Do you have any particular worries about your baby?
1 Yes
2 No
3 Other _____
8 Don't know

If yes please explain: _____
_____

24. How are you feeding your baby now?
1 Breast
2 Bottle
3 Bottle and breast
4 Other (please explain)

_____
_____

25. How much help did you have with feeding from the hospital staff?
1 A lot
2 Some
3 Not enough
4 None
5 None, but didn't want any
6 Other _____
8 Don't know

26. Do you feel that you had any problems with feeding that hospital staff could have helped with?
1 Yes
2 No
3 Didn't have any problems
4 Other _____
8 Don't know

27. What is the date you completed this form? _____/_____/_____

SURVEY NO. [   ]

THIS PAGE IS FOR YOU TO ADD ANY FURTHER NOTES OR COMMENTS.
PLEASE TELL US ANYTHING YOU THINK IS IMPORTANT.

THANK YOU VERY MUCH FOR YOUR HELP.

Index